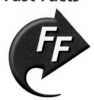

Fast Facts

Fast Facts:
Religion and Medicine

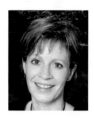

Deborah CM Boyle MD MRCOG DFFP
Locum Consultant
Department of Obstetrics and Gynaecology
Royal Free Hampstead NHS Trust
London, UK

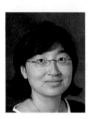

Men-Jean Lee MD FACOG
Associate Professor
Department of Obstetrics,
Gynecology & Reproductive Sciences
Yale University School of Medicine
New Haven, USA

Declaration of Independence
This book is as balanced and as practical as we can make it.
Ideas for improvement are always welcome: feedback@fastfacts.com

✝ HEALTH PRESS

Fast Facts: Religion and Medicine
First published January 2008

Text © 2008 Deborah CM Boyle, Men-Jean Lee
© 2008 in this edition Health Press Limited
Health Press Limited, Elizabeth House, Queen Street, Abingdon,
Oxford OX14 3LN, UK
Tel: +44 (0)1235 523233
Fax: +44 (0)1235 523238

Book orders can be placed by telephone or via the website.
For regional distributors or to order via the website, please go to:
www.fastfacts.com
For telephone orders, please call +44 (0)1752 202301 (UK and Europe),
1 800 247 6553 (USA, toll free), +1 419 281 1802 (Americas) or
+61 (0)2 9351 6173 (Asia–Pacific).

Fast Facts is a trademark of Health Press Limited.

The publisher and the authors have made every effort to ensure the accuracy of this
book, but cannot accept responsibility for any errors or omissions.

For all drugs, please consult the product labeling approved in your country for
prescribing information.

A CIP record for this title is available from the British Library.

ISBN: 978-1-903734-94-0

Boyle, DCM (Deborah)
Fast Facts: Religion and Medicine/
Deborah CM Boyle, Men-Jean Lee

Typesetting and page layout by Zed, Oxford, UK.
Printed by Fine Print (Services) Ltd, Oxford, UK.

Text printed with vegetable inks on biodegradable and
recyclable paper manufactured from sustainable forests.

Low emissions
during production

Low
chlorine

Sustainable
forests

Introduction

Despite living in a multicultural, multi-ethnic society, it is possible to have very little knowledge and understanding of the broad range of cultures and religions within it. Lack of knowledge may lead to misunderstandings and a failure to provide for the needs of others. This is particularly true in health services where a little knowledge may greatly enhance the quality of care on offer, avoid unintended offence and enrich the interaction between patient and care provider.

Various books have been written about the care of dying patients or about one religious group in particular, but none so far has embraced the major world religions in the context of general healthcare, including other health-related practices that may be confined to smaller groups. It is clear from talking with colleagues in family practice, nursing, midwifery and other hospital specialties that a book which helped them to better understand their patients' cultural and religious beliefs would be very valuable.

This book provides an overview of the major world religions and an introduction to the variable expression of beliefs within them and how they relate to healthcare. It is not, by any means, comprehensive, although there are suggestions for further reading. It is written from the perspective of two people interested in the lives, beliefs and wellbeing of others rather than by adherents of each faith, and this is reflected in the text. Throughout the book the notation BCE (before Common Era) and CE (Common Era) replace the terms BC (Before Christ) and AD (Anno Domini) as non-Christian religions do not use this terminology.

Understanding the cultural practices and religious backgrounds of the patients we serve can improve our communication with both patients and concerned family members, and enrich the sensitive healthcare that we seek to provide. When we integrate medical practice with consideration of the faith of the individual patient, we are providing personalized care that will go a long way to improving the medical outcome.

1   Buddhism

There are approximately 390 million
Buddhists worldwide representing
about 6% of the world's population.
Buddhism originated in Northern
India and is a way of life that has
been followed for around 2500 years.
The symbol of Buddhism is the
Dharma Wheel which represents the
Buddha's teaching of the path to
enlightenment.

Buddhists hope to release themselves from desire and reach
enlightenment or nirvana by escaping the cycle of birth and rebirth into
which man is tied through desire. Through the teachings of the Buddha,
followers hope to develop the qualities of wisdom, non-violence and
compassion. Although Buddhists believe in a higher plane, they do not
generally refer to it as God and some prefer to think of their beliefs as a
philosophy of life rather than a religion.

Siddharta Gautama is the historic founder of Buddhism. He was born
in 560 BCE in North Eastern India into a life of great privilege. His
mother died 7 days after his birth, which has led to the belief that a
woman who gives birth to a Buddha cannot serve any other purpose.
The young prince was raised by his aunt. When he grew up, he married
Gopa and they called their first son Rahula (meaning 'chains'), which
reflected how the young prince felt imprisoned by his lifestyle. One day,
he escaped from the palace and had four experiences.

- He saw a frail old man and witnessed how old age destroys memory,
  strength and beauty. He had not previously encountered old age.
- He saw a sick person racked with pain and was shocked to see, for
  the first time, so much pain and suffering.
- He saw weeping mourners at a funeral procession and was disturbed
  by the distress of death, which he had not encountered before.
- He saw a holy man with an alms bowl who was contented and happy.

These experiences led Siddharta to the conclusion that all of life's pleasures are ephemeral and worthless. He wished to find true knowledge and left the palace in order to find it. He tried many different ways of finding enlightenment including joining the monks, undertaking yoga and living in extreme poverty, but to no avail. He then sat under a bodhi tree to meditate, and enlightenment finally came to him in three stages over three nights: on the first night, all of his previous lives passed before him; on the second night, the cycle of birth and rebirth and the laws that govern it were revealed to him; and on the third night, he came to understand the Four Noble Truths.

- Suffering is universal.
- The origin of suffering is human desire.
- The cessation of suffering can be achieved.
- There is a path to the cessation of suffering.

He realized that if human craving ceased, suffering would also cease. In this way, he became the Buddha or 'the enlightened one'. Following this, Buddha was asked by the high God, Brahma, to help others find enlightenment, which he did for the remainder of his life.

Sects

There are two predominant forms of Buddhism: Theravada and Mahayana. Theravada is the path usually followed by monks, but most Buddhists follow the path of Mahayana.

Theravada Buddhists. Theravada Buddhism is practiced in Sri Lanka, Myanmar (formerly Burma), Thailand and other parts of South East Asia. An important emphasis within Theravada Buddhism is that the Buddha was only a man and one in a succession of Buddhas, but that enlightenment may be attained by following his teachings.

The Theravada Buddhists are further divided into two groups: the monks or nuns and householders. The monks and nuns or *bhikkus* rely entirely on others for the provision of food and clothing. They beg for alms from the householders, but are only allowed to do so before midday. By being free of domestic duties and devoting much time to meditation, the *bhikkus* stand the best chance of enlightenment. It is believed that only monks and nuns can truly attain enlightenment.

Householders make gifts to the monks and nuns in the hope of a better rebirth in the next cycle.

Mahayana Buddhists also believe that there is more than one Buddha, but they regard Siddharta Gautama as superhuman. This form of Buddhism offers more ways to enlightenment than Theravada based on the three principles established by following the Buddha's teachings.

- One does not have to reach enlightenment through one's own efforts alone; there are Bodhisattvas on earth who have already attained enlightenment, but remain here in order to help others do the same.
- Anything may be used in the journey to enlightenment including wood-carvings and the chanting of mantras.
- The community of monks and nuns known as the *sangha* may help a person.

Mahayana Buddhism is subdivided into many schools and is the main form of Buddhism found in China, Japan, Tibet, Mongolia, Korea and Nepal.

Other sects. A further branch of Buddhism is that of the Friends of the Western Buddhist Order, which has branches in the UK and USA, and Order members elsewhere, such as India. Due to geographic and cultural differences, this branch of Buddhism has adapted itself to a more Western lifestyle and is the basis for much of the information regarding health and general lifestyle in this Chapter.

Of the various forms of Buddhism in Japan, one of the most curious is Zen Buddhism. This teaches that one must get beyond words in order to achieve enlightenment. This has led to monks spending many years meditating on a single word or sentence, or a puzzle called a *koan* that has no answer such as 'what is the sound of one hand clapping?'.

Scriptures

The scriptures of the Theravada Buddhists are called the 'Pali Canon' and consist of three parts relating to the monks and nuns, the various discourses given by the Buddha and an analysis of the discourses. They are written in the language of Pali and, where possible, are still read in that language.

The Mahayana scriptures were written in Sanskrit and much of their content is contained within the Pali Canon. Other books have been added and these additional writings are considered to be the authoritative 'word' of the Buddha. Tibetan Buddhists believe that many scriptures were hidden until the time was right for them to be understood. They are still being revealed and one of the best known is *The Tibetan Book of the Dead*.

The Buddha taught that the vision of enlightenment, which was revealed to him, could be achieved by others if they believed the Four Noble Truths (see page 8) and followed the Eightfold Path or 'middle way' in order to overcome desire and thus end human suffering. The Eightfold Path aims for a life between asceticism and hedonism, and the eight different elements can be regarded as being like the spokes of a wheel:

- right understanding of the Four Noble Truths
- right thoughts leading to love for all living things, even the most humble
- right speech, which must be pure, noble and well-intentioned
- right action involving moral behavior, being considerate to others and showing kindness to all living creatures
- right livelihood: a Buddhist monk must not earn a living from anything that involves violence or from following their religion, and Buddhist monks must be kept by the community
- right effort to banish all evil thoughts
- right mindfulness involving constant awareness of the needs of others
- right concentration using meditation, which allows a person to become inwardly calm and at peace with themselves and the world.

In addition to the Four Noble Truths and the Eightfold Path, the Five Precepts provide moral guidance to the life of a Buddhist. These are:

- avoid taking life or harming any living thing
- avoid taking anything which is not given
- avoid all sexual misconduct
- avoid all unworthy speech such as gossiping, lying and idle speculation
- avoid drugs and alcohol as these affect the mind and judgment.

All living things are in a cycle of birth and rebirth until they reach nirvana, or the place of coolness, where the fire of desire has been extinguished. Buddha taught that all life is in a constant state of flux and that nothing is permanent, even the soul. In this respect Buddhism and Hinduism are different, as Hindus believe that there is a permanent soul or *atman*.

Worship

Although Buddha was a teacher rather than a God, Buddhist worship still involves paying homage to images of the Buddha. Worship may take place in a public temple or at a private shrine in the home. Much of Buddhist worship is quiet, involving offerings and meditation, but teaching is also a component.

Offerings may include flowers as a reminder of the impermanence of life, incense as a reminder of the lasting fragrance of the Buddha's teachings and light to dispel the darkness. Mahayana Buddhists may make a sevenfold offering to the Buddha, which is commonly symbolized by seven bowls of water that may be used for drinking, bathing or foot-washing.

Meditation is an important part of Buddhism and is used to rid the mind of impure thoughts and distractions to allow a calm and wise state to develop. There are different styles of meditation, but they are all designed to bring tranquility to the mind and with it, insight. Mantras may be chanted to assist with meditation and some believe that this can lead to a higher form of consciousness by the generation of vibrations within the body.

There are no prayers in Buddhism, because there is no-one to offer them to. Instead, Buddhists pledge to live their lives in the right way, modeled on the life and teachings of the Buddha.

Festivals

Festivals and celebrations are not a prominent part of Buddhism, since the Buddha's teachings say that people should not attach spiritual significance to such matters. What is important is the state of mind of those celebrating the festival. There are festivals within Buddhism, which vary from country to country, and according to the particular strand of Buddhism. The calendar is determined by the cycles of the moon and all festival days occur at full moon, which is regarded as auspicious by Buddhists.

- Buddha Day in May celebrates the enlightenment of the Buddha.
- Dharma day, which is usually in July, recalls the Buddha's teachings.
- Padma Sambhava day in September celebrates a semi-mythical figure responsible for taking Buddhism to Tibet.
- Sangha day in November celebrates the community of people.
- Parinirvana day in February recalls the death of the Buddha.

Marriage

In some Buddhist sects, monks and nuns are permitted to marry and have children. Japanese and Korean monks may get married, and Theravada monks may leave the monastery to become married. However, Chinese, Taiwanese and Vietnamese monks take a vow of celibacy.

Dress

There are no restrictions regarding dress in Buddhism, except for those who are part of a monastic Order who wear robes. In some parts of the world, robes are saffron colored, but in others, such as Tibet, they are maroon.

Food and drink

The principle of non-violence informs every aspect of the life of a Buddhist and many extend this to their diet. Buddhists commonly eat a vegetarian diet and avoid eating animals that have been killed for food.

There are certain parts of the world where following a vegetarian diet would be difficult or even ill-advised owing to the shortage of good quality vegetables. One such place is Tibet, where the climate and topography make the growing of crops very difficult.

Buddhist monks in some parts of the world must survive on whatever is put into their alms bowls and for some this makes eating meat acceptable. For others, acceptance of meat is dependent on the meat not having come from an animal killed specifically for the purpose of food production.

Contraception and reproduction

There is no general agreement among Buddhists as to when consciousness develops in a potential human being, but the process of producing a new human life is regarded as the coming together of sperm, egg and consciousness. In general, abortion is discouraged, but it is not strictly prohibited; Buddhists in the West would generally take the view that it was not for anyone else to stand in judgment of another who felt that she had just cause to seek an abortion. Opinions and practice vary according to country and cultural background.

There are no restrictions on the use of contraceptives or the methods used. Some methods, such as intrauterine contraceptive devices, work partly by causing the shedding of any fertilized eggs very early on. For this reason, some women and couples may prefer to use another method where the possibility of shedding a fertilized egg does not occur.

Death

Of all stages in life, death is the most important to a Buddhist. The certain knowledge that death will come to us all, and that we should prepare for it and make the most of life until it comes, underpins Buddhist philosophy.

Buddhists believe that consciousness continues after the death of a body, but it is difficult to describe the exact form it takes. The general concept is that the consciousness will be reborn into another human form and inform the actions and emotions of the person into whom it has been reborn. Events that occur in a person's life are believed to result, in part, from the consciousness of that person's previous lives. This has led to the development of ancestor worship by Chinese Buddhists. It is common practice for people to create family shrines to pray to their ancestors for support, serve food to the ancestral spirits during auspicious occasions and burn symbols of paper money for the ancestors to use in their other lives.

There is no God in Buddhism and therefore no-one to judge the life of a person when they die. The destiny of the consciousness is therefore not determined by a supreme being and it is not, as commonly thought, determined by a person's actions during life (e.g. non-beneficial actions will not lead to rebirth as a lower life form, such as an earthworm).

The various strands of Buddhism have different practices with regard to death. Tibetan Buddhists, for example, believe that there is a stage between death and rebirth, which lasts for 49 days and is known as the *bardo*. During this time, fellow Buddhists read *The Tibetan Book of the Dead* to the dead person and encourage them to move towards the light and the Buddhas. The belief is that the dead person experiences the pull of both these things but, because it is both strong and overwhelming, they need courage to embrace it rather than to shy away.

The dead body is not treated in any specific way, but tends to be left uncovered so that others may meditate next to it and pay their respects. Funeral services are usually conducted by ordained members of the Order or may be conducted by a friend of the dead person. The funeral service will include meditation, and reflection and celebration of the life of the deceased. As the funeral service may be quite lengthy, it is not uncommon, at least in Western countries, for this to take place away from the crematorium or graveyard. Most Buddhists are cremated, though some may prefer to be buried on ecological grounds or simply due to personal preference. Chinese Buddhists may use feng shui to determine where the deceased should be buried.

Key points – Buddhism

- Buddhism was founded around 2500 years ago in North Eastern India by Siddharta Gautama who became the Buddha or 'the enlightened one'.
- Buddhism is founded on the 'Four Noble Truths' designed to relieve human suffering, overcome desire and produce a state of 'enlightenment'.
- Buddhists are usually vegetarian, although some will eat meat from an animal that has not been killed specifically for food.
- Abortion is generally discouraged but is not strictly prohibited.
- There are no restrictions on the use of contraception or the method used.
- Of all aspects of existence, death and the rituals attached to it are the most important.

2 Christianity

Christianity is the world's largest religion. It is followed by an estimated 33% of the world's population and there are thought to be about 2.1 billion Christians worldwide. In Africa, there are now more Christians than Muslims; Muslims tend to be concentrated in the northern half of the continent, but Christians predominate in central and southern countries.

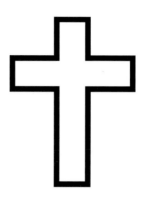

Elsewhere, countries that have previously been dominated by another faith, such as the traditionally Buddhist Taiwan, are experiencing a gradual conversion to a Christian majority.

Christians believe that Jesus Christ was the Son of God and the Son of Man – human and yet divine – whose death and resurrection freed the world from sin. The Christian cross is the symbol of the crucifixion of Jesus and the empty cross shows that he has risen again.

Jesus was born a Jew in Palestine just over 2000 years ago. He traveled around gathering followers, interpreting Jewish law, providing people with a code by which to live their lives and performing miracles. Initially, he preached in Jewish synagogues, but opposition meant he ultimately had to teach his disciples and followers elsewhere. Eventually, Jesus was arrested and charged with incitement to rebellion by the Romans, and of blasphemy and opposing Jewish law by religious leaders. He predicted his own death at a meal, known as the Last Supper, with his disciples to celebrate the Jewish feast of Passover. During this meal, Jesus used bread and wine to signify his body and blood, which were about to be given up, and told the disciples that this would be done in order to save the world from sin. At church services during Holy Communion or the Eucharist, bread and wine are shared in memory of the Last Supper and as an acknowledgment of what Christ's death represents. Jesus was ultimately put to death on a cross under the instructions of Pontius Pilate, the Roman Governor at the time. He died a slow and painful death, and his body was placed in a tomb. Three days later, the body had disappeared from the tomb and Jesus appeared to his followers that day and twice thereafter. The death and resurrection of Jesus are remembered the world over by Christians on Good Friday and Easter Day. Jesus made one final appearance when he was seen ascending into heaven 40 days after the resurrection; this is celebrated by some Christians on Ascension Day.

The Christian church was effectively 'born' on the day of Pentecost. (This is also the day when Jews celebrate the gift of the Torah to Moses on Mount Sinai.) It was on this day following the death of Jesus that the disciples heard a rushing noise and saw flames resting on each of them. This fulfilled the prophecy of Jesus that they would receive the Holy Spirit from God. The disciples subsequently preached the message of Jesus as he had foretold. One of the disciples, Peter, preached that there were four fundamental beliefs.

- Jesus was the Messiah.
- The Messiah died and was resurrected.
- Those who were sorry for their sins would be forgiven by God.
- Jesus sits at the right hand of God in heaven.

The apostle Paul did much to further the message of the early church and to welcome Jews and gentiles in many parts. His letters to people he met and his writings to encourage them in their beliefs form part of the Christian Bible.

Sects

Most Christians are Roman Catholic (1.2 billion), but there are also large numbers of Protestants (427 million) and Eastern Orthodox Christians (240 million).

The Christian religion is broadly divided, geographically, into East and West, reflecting a schism that occurred hundreds of years ago. In the East (e.g. Russia, Greece, Armenia, Ukraine), Orthodox beliefs prevail. In the West (USA and Europe), Roman Catholic and Anglican churches are more widespread. Worldwide, however, Christians are divided between many more denominations.

Other Christian groups whose beliefs differ more widely, such as the Jehovah's Witnesses, Seventh-day Adventists and Mormons, are discussed separately in Chapter 8.

Scripture

The Holy Bible is the holy book of Christians, which some believe was divinely inspired and others use as a guide to everyday living. There are two parts to the Holy Bible: the Old Testament and the New Testament. The Old Testament contains 'books' derived from the Jewish scriptures, and the New Testament contains Christian writings and includes the four Gospels, Acts of the Apostles, 21 letters or Epistles mostly written by Paul and the book of Revelation.

Worship

The largest gatherings for Christian worship take place in churches on Sundays, the Christian Sabbath, though worship takes place every day of the week. Although churches vary in design from very large and ornate to small and simple, some features are common to most of them.

The emphasis and style of worship varies between denominations. For example, in the Presbyterian Church, worship takes place in rather bare buildings and is accompanied by little music, preferring to concentrate on 'the Word'. Other churches may have ornate buildings and incorporate beautiful music in the form of gospel choirs or congregations singing traditional hymns. More modern churches, however, may opt for folk songs sung with guitars. Roman Catholic and Anglo-Catholic churches often use incense.

The structure of a Service of Worship may vary between denominations, but will generally involve readings from the Old and New Testaments of the Bible and a reading from one of the Gospels (of which there are four) on a cyclical basis. Prayers will be said, some of which are 'prescribed' and others that are more free-ranging; again, this will depend on the particular denomination.

The inclusion, or otherwise, of the sharing of bread and wine, is determined by denomination and will usually be included in all Roman or Anglo-Catholic Services, but may form part of only some services for other groups.

Pilgrimage

Christian pilgrims often visit sites where miracles are said to have occurred. One of the best known is Lourdes, France, where people go in the hope that their prayers may be answered. Some Christians make pilgrimages to the Vatican in Rome, Italy, and to Bethlehem, Palestine, which was the birthplace of Jesus.

Festivals

The four major 'seasons' in the Christian calendar are those of Advent, Christmas, Lent and Easter.

Advent. The season of Advent is the four Sundays and intervening weeks leading up to Christmas Day on 25th December, when the Western Church celebrates the birth of Christ or 'the embodiment of God's word in human form'. The Orthodox Church celebrates Christmas on 6th January or the Epiphany, which is the day when the Western church celebrates the visit of the three wise men to the newborn Jesus.

Christmas. The season of Christmas embraces the period from 25th December to 2nd February, with the latter date commemorating the presentation of Jesus Christ in the Temple.

Lent is the 40-day period (excluding Sundays) before Easter. During this time, many Christians will abstain from something that they normally enjoy as an act of symbolism to remind them of the fasting Jesus undertook before beginning his ministry. In the USA, this abstinence typically consists of not eating meat on Fridays and, in recognition, many restaurants provide fish dishes.

The day before the start of Lent is Mardi Gras (which literally translates as 'fat Tuesday') when butter and eggs were traditionally used up before Lent; it is also known as Shrove Tuesday or pancake day in the UK. It is cause for celebration before the start of the Lenten fasts. The first day of Lent is Ash Wednesday, when Catholics attend Mass and receive the sign of the cross on their foreheads with the ashes from the burnt dried palms from the previous year's Palm Sunday.

Lent culminates in Holy Week, which starts on Palm Sunday. Palm Sunday commemorates the triumphant entry of Jesus into the city of Jerusalem when people paved the streets with palm leaves. It is followed 4 days later by Maundy Thursday, which remembers Jesus washing the feet of his disciples as a mark of his humility. The following day is Good Friday when the death of Jesus on the cross is remembered. This is the most solemn day in the Christian calendar and many churches have vigils between noon and 3 PM to recall the particular time when Jesus died. In some churches, the event is commemorated by a re-enactment of the events leading to the Crucifixion known as 'the Passion of Christ'. The following Sunday is Easter Day when the resurrection of Jesus is celebrated.

Easter. Originally, the feast of Easter coincided with the Jewish feast of Passover. By decree this was changed so that Easter would fall on the first Sunday after the spring full moon. The calendars of the Christian churches in the East and West are different, and the day on which Easter is celebrated may vary by up to 5 weeks.

Easter is traditionally celebrated with a feast of lamb and other meats that have been abstained from during the period of Lent, and children participate in Easter egg hunts in both the USA and UK.

Pentecost. The Feast of Pentecost is 7 weeks after Easter. It recalls the visit of the Holy Spirit to the disciples and the birth of the church. As with the Passover, this festival is a 'Christianized' version of another Jewish festival, Shavuot, when Moses was given the Torah by God. A tradition developed in which converts to Christianity would wear white clothes and be baptized on the day of the Pentecost; hence the alternative name of Whitsunday (or White Sunday).

Other festivals throughout the year are not celebrated by all Christians and are not public holidays. They commemorate events such as the Annunciation to Mary, the mother of Jesus, that she would give birth to the new Messiah, and Ascension Day when Jesus finally left the earth and ascended to heaven.

Sacraments and rites of passage

Sacraments are ceremonies or rituals that represent the ministry of Jesus. They are at the heart of worship in the Roman Catholic and Orthodox churches, as well as many Anglican and Episcopalian churches. Most Protestant churches celebrate the sacraments of baptism and communion. The Quaker, Salvation Army and other churches do not celebrate any sacraments; though they have services for ordination, marriage and confirmation, they do not regard them as sacraments.

Roman Catholics and other Christians celebrate the seven sacraments or 'mysteries' as they are known by the Orthodox Church. Together with communion, they comprise baptism, confession or reconciliation, confirmation, marriage, holy orders and anointing of the sick and dying.

Holy Baptism (or Christening) is the acknowledgment that a person is a Christian and cleanses the soul of sin. It is not a naming ceremony, as is often thought. In Roman Catholic, Orthodox and Anglican churches, babies and small children are often baptized and it is seen as the introduction of the child into the family faith. The Christening is also the opportunity for the parents to name godparents (other close members of the family and friends) to look after the religious development of the child.

Baptism may be especially important if the baby or child is sick, particularly if the parents are Roman Catholic and believe that the child's soul is in peril if the child dies without being baptized. In these circumstances, offering to contact a priest or suggesting that the parents may wish to do so is appropriate. In the case of stillbirth, attendant physicians or nurses may perform a respectful blessing/baptism immediately after delivery, regardless of the gestational age of the fetus, at the parents' request.

Holy Communion. The service in which bread and wine is shared is known by different names. It is called the Mass by Roman Catholics, the Eucharist by Anglicans, the Lord's Supper by Baptists and the Divine Feast by Orthodox Christians. The bread represents the body of Christ and is often represented by a thin rice paper wafer. The wine represents the blood of Christ and is sipped from a shared goblet.

The First Holy Communion taken by a young person in the Roman and Anglo-Catholic Churches following a period of instruction is cause for celebration.

Confession is the confessing of and absolution from sins, but is being replaced by the 'sacrament of reconciliation'. 'Confessions' are heard by a priest who will then suggest some means of absolution by the saying of prayers, possibly with reparation and an undertaking to try to avoid repeating mistakes.

In Catholic and some Anglican churches, confessions are made in a confessional, behind closed doors in booths separating the priest from the penitent. The frequency with which Confession is undertaken varies according to the individual. Children may begin this sacrament after receiving the First Holy Communion.

Confirmation takes place following several years of continued religious education. During the ceremony, a young person or adult becomes a full member of the church and confirms their vows as a Christian. Children are typically confirmed at around 10–12 years of age, though confirmation may take place at any age thereafter for any person wishing to become a full member of the Church. Traditionally, boys and girls are dressed in white and the day is an opportunity for a family and community celebration.

Marriage. In the Roman Catholic Church, the marriage ceremony involves a full Mass with Holy Communion (the Nuptial Mass). Catholic and other Orthodox Christian churches may require a couple to undergo several months of premarital religious counseling (known as 'pre-Cana' in the USA) before the priest will agree to perform the marriage rites.

Holy Orders is the dedication of a person to a religious life and the ordination by the laying on of hands with prayer of those able to administer the sacraments, namely, priests, bishops, archbishops and others. In Protestant churches, ministers, preachers, deacons and other volunteers can lead services for worship.

Anointing of the Sick, which is also known as extreme unction or last rites, is the anointing of a sick person with holy oil. In the Roman Catholic faith this will also include Holy Communion given by a priest.

Family

As with most faiths, family, marriage and the raising of children within a family is regarded as important. Divorce is discouraged, but the breakdown of relationships is regarded as a sad fact of life by most Christians. Some groups take a stronger line on this, particularly those in the Orthodox Christian and Catholic faiths. More progressive Christian denominations accept same-sex families and blended families into their congregations.

Dress

Most Christians are not recognizable by their attire. Priests wear clothes that signify their occupation, at least when they are ministering to their parishioners. In Western churches, they wear a plain shirt and trousers or skirt in a shade appropriate to their status within the church. A white band or 'dog collar' is worn around the neck and tucked under the adapted shirt collar. Orthodox priests usually wear a long black garment that buttons down the front and a tall hat.

Catholic Nuns wear a habit consisting of a uniform dress and a wimple, which is a head covering that drapes at the back like a veil. Modern nuns, however, may not wear the wimple, particularly if their vocation involves working in a hospital or as a teacher. Alternatively, they may wear a combination of uniform appropriate to their occupation and the wimple (e.g. nursing and midwifery staff).

In Mediterranean countries, Catholic widows tend to wear black clothes all or most of the time. Rosary beads, pendants in the shape of the cross and medallions of a patron saint may also be worn as symbols of their faith.

Some Christian denominations are instantly recognizable by their dress and demeanor. Amish families wear old-fashioned clothes, and girls and women will not cut their hair and will wear headscarves. Plymouth Brethren female members also wear white or blue headscarves over long hair.

Food and drink

Most denominations do not have any specific dietary restrictions. However, devout Roman Catholics will not eat meat on Good Friday.

Fasting is uncommon within the Christian faith, though some devout Roman Catholics prefer to fast each Sunday before taking Communion and many Catholics/Anglo-Catholics will abstain from something that they normally enjoy during the season of Lent before Easter. This is in recognition of the fast for 40 days and nights that Jesus was said to have undertaken in the wilderness while being tempted by the devil. As with other faiths where any form of fasting is practiced, it is designed to help reflective thought and to focus on prayer.

Contraception and reproduction

Some Catholics find any form of contraception unacceptable, including the use of condoms or oral contraceptive pills, though this attitude is becoming rarer. Permanent tubal sterilization is also prohibited by the Catholic faith and is unavailable at Catholic hospitals.

Other groups, who consider that a person has a soul from the moment of fertilization of the human egg, find only some forms of contraception unacceptable. They consider using any method of contraception that promotes the shedding of a fertilized egg or abortion as murder and a spiritual crime. Intrauterine contraceptive devices (IUCDs or IUDs) may therefore be unacceptable, with the possible exception of the levonorgestrel-containing intrauterine system (LNG-IUS; Mirena®), which works in a different way. Standard IUCDs make fertilization less likely, but also make the uterine lining hostile to any egg that may have been fertilized, and it is this potential deliberate shedding of the fertilized egg that is a source of contention for some. The LNG-IUS, however, makes fertilization less likely by thickening the cervical mucus and thus providing a physical barrier to sperm entering the uterus, and also impeding the process of fertilization by any sperm that may have entered. It also thins the uterine lining to prevent implantation of any fertilized egg. The uncertainties of how likely an egg is to be fertilized in the presence of an IUCD or the LNG-IUS mean that women who are strictly opposed to methods that prevent implantation of an embryo will not find these devices acceptable.

Although some Christians, along with followers of some other religions, may have strong feelings about termination of pregnancy on 'social' grounds, they may be prepared to consider it when antenatal diagnosis reveals that a woman is carrying a baby affected by a serious congenital condition. The boundaries for any individual or couple are a personal matter and it should never be assumed that, simply because a person is a Roman Catholic or of any other denomination, that they will be opposed to termination of pregnancy in any circumstances.

Sexuality

Given that marriage and the raising of children within a 'traditional' family structure are highly valued in the Christian faith, homosexuality provokes a variety of reactions. Despite a general increase in tolerance of homosexuality, gay relationships and even gay clergy in some quarters, the subject is currently the focus of fierce debate and difference of opinion within the worldwide Anglican Communion. Indeed, there is a significant threat to the unity of the worldwide Anglican Communion over the issue of appointing an openly gay bishop in the USA, with some groups suggesting that they will break away from the main body unless the appointment is revoked.

Death

Last rites are important to many Christians and a priest may be called to say prayers with a dying person and administer Holy Communion and/or a blessing. Christians believe that death is not the end, but rather the passing of the soul into heaven to be united with God. Roman Catholics believe that the soul does not pass directly to heaven, but spends a period of time in purgatory where it is spiritually cleansed. Prayers are offered to shorten the time of the soul in purgatory. The way in which funeral services are conducted varies according to denomination. In general, whether a body is cremated or buried is left to personal preference. Memorial services may be held some time after the funeral to give thanks for the life of the deceased.

Traditionally, Roman Catholic funerals start with the body being laid at the home of the deceased, where prayers are said in an all-night vigil (also known as a wake). More commonly nowadays, the body will be laid either in the church or in the chapel of rest at the funeral parlor. This gives immediate family members an opportunity to visit the body and receive visits and words of condolences from friends and family members over 1–3 days, depending on the wishes of the deceased or family members. The room may contain floral wreaths or arrangements and pictures of the deceased with their friends and families. The grieving family and guests are typically dressed in black for mourning.

During Roman Catholic and Anglican funerals, the service comprises prayers, hymns and a eulogy, and those present are reminded that the soul of the deceased is being commended directly to God.

Orthodox Christians believe that there is no difference between the living and the dead, and all are part of the Kingdom of God. Following the death of a believer, the body is washed and dressed in new clothes and placed in an open coffin. Icons of Jesus, Mary and John the Baptist are placed on the forehead of the body, which is then covered with a linen cloth to symbolize Christ's protection. The coffin lid is not closed until the service is over.

In the USA, once the funeral service has finished, close friends and immediate family members form a funeral procession by following the hearse in their cars with their headlights on. They then drive around the neighborhood in which the deceased lived and other places with special meaning, before ending at the cemetery.

Burials are typically very private events. In Europe, funerals may take different forms. The cremation or burial may be preceded by a church service with a procession of funeral cars to move the coffin and mourners from one place to another, or may be conducted entirely at the crematorium.

Although funerals are solemn occasions for most Christians, it is becoming more common in the USA for the deceased to request that their friends and families celebrate their lives with parties, such as ten-pin bowling, magicians, and rock-and-roll guitar music.

Autopsies are generally acceptable to Christian families if clinically indicated.

Key points – Christianity

- Christianity was founded just over 2000 years ago.
- Christians believe that Jesus Christ was the Son of God and the Son of Man – human and yet divine.
- There are many groups under the umbrella term 'Christian', but the largest is the Roman Catholic Church followed by the Protestant groups and then Orthodox Christians.
- There is widespread variation in the interpretation of biblical laws and also in expression of faith.
- Some Catholics find any form of contraception unacceptable, and permanent tubal sterilization is prohibited by the Catholic faith.
- Many Christians have strong feelings about abortion, but the boundaries for individuals or couples may vary.

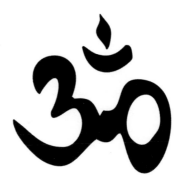

Hinduism is the world's third largest religion after Christianity and Islam. There are over 1 billion Hindus worldwide representing approximately 13% of the world's population. Although India is the origin and spiritual home of the Hindu faith, Hindus have settled in 160 countries throughout the world with around 1 million in the UK and 800 000 in the USA.

The Hindu faith is also the oldest in the world, but is probably the most difficult to understand. Unlike the other major world religions, it does not have a single founder or prophet nor does it have a single book of scripture. It is a religion that has evolved over time and has many different sects – the Shaivas, Jains, Swaminarayanis and Vaishnavas to name but a few – each with their own beliefs and methods of expression.

The name 'Hindu' derives from Sanskrit literature and was originally a geographic term indicating a person from India. Since the way of life and religious beliefs could not be separated and there was no special name for the religion, the term Hindu eventually came to have religious significance.

To be a Hindu is not merely to observe religious rituals and ceremonies, but to live a life that is a synthesis of worship, morals, a code of conduct and duty, based on the laws of nature, in the hope that the soul (*atman*) may be released from its cycle of birth and rebirth (reincarnation), and be finally reunited with God in salvation (*moksha*). Non-violence is a philosophy that runs through all aspects of Hindu life, and the idea that all living creatures have a soul and that their right to live should be respected is expressed in various ways, such as peaceful living and vegetarianism.

In India, a divisive 'caste' system still exists, despite the efforts of several reformers, whereby a person is born into a certain class and may not move out of it. Caste determines the kind of jobs people are allowed to do and their marriage prospects; the Brahmin or priest caste is the highest ranking and the untouchable caste is the lowest. It is now illegal in India to enforce the caste system and temples are now open to all. Theoretically at least, a person is now free to marry whomever he or she pleases, but in practice even the most liberal of parents want their children to marry within the same caste, though these rigid barriers are slowly breaking down.

Scripture

The Vedas are ancient texts which define truth for Hindus. Hindus believe that the texts were passed directly from God to scholars and for hundreds, possibly thousands, of years they were passed on orally. There are four Vedas, each with a further four parts. Vedas are sometimes known as *shrutis*, which means 'for hearing'.

Other texts are known as *smritis*, meaning 'what is remembered'. The Bhagavad Gita or 'Song of the Lord' forms part of these texts and is part of the world's longest poem. The Ramayana is another of the *smritis* and tells the story of Prince Rama. It is regarded as a story of good overcoming evil, though there have been a number of interpretations.

Worship

Perhaps the most confusing issue for non-Hindus to understand is the concept of God in the Hindu faith. While there may appear to be many Gods, in fact there is only one God with many representations in the form of people, animals or a hybrid of both and many different names, all of which reflect different facets of the deity. In both personal and public worship, idols of these forms are used by practicing Hindus as an aid to worship to provide a tangible, inspirational reminder of the presence of God and something on which to bestow praise. Hindus believe that God is everywhere and in everything, so anything that helps a person to visualize God for themselves is acceptable as a focus and form of worship. Hindu

worship takes several forms.

Personal prayer at home is regarded as very important. Hindu homes usually contain a statue of the family's chosen form(s) of God. Offerings of fruit, flowers, perfumed substances, incense and candles together with prayers may be made to this image of God on a daily basis and each of the offerings has its own significance. There is also a strong sense of appreciation for nature in Hindu prayers as an acknowledgment of the importance of the various elements for living.

Yoga (from the Sanskrit word *yuj* meaning to meet or come together) is another form of personal worship. It represents the joining of a person with God and reflects the threefold nature of a person: spiritual, intellectual and mental. Hindus believe that the soul of a person becomes united with God when meditating or praying. There are different forms of yoga, but all have the same aim – to unite the soul with God through physical preparation, breathing and detachment from worldly distractions. Yoga has become very popular in the West as a form of exercise and physical conditioning, but this is only part of what yoga is about.

Communal worship led by Hindu priests and involving reading from the 'living' scriptures, takes place in temples. Hindu temples or *mandirs* are beautiful structures built according to strict rules about where they should be placed and how they should be constructed. Every part of a temple is sacred, which is why footwear must be removed before entering. Temples have several purposes:

- to house a religious atmosphere and engender pious thoughts in the minds of those who visit them
- to generate a feeling of calm and mental wellbeing
- to encourage communal worship, which creates religious purity and solidarity in the community and reduces tension and conflict by encouraging people to live together harmoniously
- to provide a house for the deity to live in splendor.

Temples are also places for education and socializing as well as for worship.

Aum. The symbol 'aum' (or 'om') is central to Hindu worship (see figure, page 27). In the Sanskrit language, the two letters 'a' and 'u' combine to form 'o', hence the two different written formats. The word aum is believed to have given rise to language and to be the best name for God. Although it is difficult to define, aum also embraces the idea that God is omnipresent, omniscient and omnipotent. Repeating the word aum is part of Hindu worship and also helps to focus the mind during meditation.

Pilgrimage

In common with other major world religions, pilgrimage is a part of Hinduism. Although it is not as obligatory as in Islam, it is considered important to undertake a pilgrimage at some point in one's life. The aims of pilgrimage are to obtain purification, visit the faith's holy places in India, develop humility and discover one's heritage. Pilgrimages may be undertaken as a vow or following a birth or death within the family.

During pilgrimage, some pilgrims may abstain from meat and alcohol to maintain purity. Once they reach the place of pilgrimage, pilgrims may attend morning and evening worship, make offerings in memory of departed ancestors and visit the family priest. They may also go to see the holy image kept in the inner sanctum of the holy place, which can involve waiting for days if many pilgrims are visiting at the same time, such as at special festivals.

Holy sites. There are many sites regarded as holy by Hindus, which may be associated with specific deities (e.g. Mathura is famous as the birthplace of Krishna) or places where significant events occurred (e.g. Kanyakumari is the site where the Goddess Paravati married Lord Shiva). The River Ganges has a special significance as it is regarded as the mother of all rivers. It is believed that if a dying person sips the water of the Ganges, his or her soul will be liberated. Similarly, it is also believed that, if a dead person is cremated on the banks of the Ganges and the ashes scattered into the river, the soul will be finally liberated from its cycle of birth and rebirth; if a person does not die within reach of the Ganges, the body may be flown thousands of miles in order for this to be achieved.

The most holy place of all is perhaps Varanasi (also known as Benares) on the banks of the river Ganges. It has a famous *mandir* or temple and many Hindus retire here in the hope of achieving liberation. It is famous for its *ghats* (steps leading down to the river) and is a favored place for both the cremation of bodies and the scattering of ashes.

Festivals

The Hindu calendar is lunar and, as a consequence, an extra month is added to the year every 4 years as each lunar month is only 29 days. In comparison, the Gregorian calendar has 30–31 days each month. The month is divided into a 'bright fortnight' and a 'dark fortnight' during the phases when the moon waxes and wanes, respectively. The days of full moon are considered very auspicious and each has a Hindu festival attached to it.

Hindu festivals are a time of great rejoicing. They mark cycles of the seasons, celebrate the harvest and commemorate important Indian national heroes. Celebration of festivals varies from community to community and according to geographic location. The dates for the festivals are fixed each year according to the lunar cycles so exact Gregorian dates cannot be given, with the exception of *Makara Sankranti*, which always falls on 14th January when the sun enters Capricorn and travels on a northward path; traveling on a northward path is believed by Hindus to be going towards God or noble direction. On this day, people may exchange colored sesame seeds or sugar grains with a pledge for only friendship to exist between them from here onwards. Traditionally, balls of sesame seeds and sugar (*til ladoos*) are given to the Brahmins and children fly kites. Any donations made on this day are thought to be particularly auspicious.

The festival of Diwali or the Festival of Lights celebrates the beginning of the new Hindu year and occurs sometime between September and November (depending on the lunar calendar). During the 5 days of the festival, lights in the form of candles, lamps and fireworks are illuminated to welcome Lakshmi, the goddess of wealth. The day after Diwali is the first day of the New Year when businesses open new account books, and friends and family meet and visit the temple.

Every 12 years (the last festival was held in 2001), 30 million people gather (the biggest gathering in the world) at one of four sites in India. At these gatherings known as *Kumbha Mela*, religious leaders preach, holy men emerge from their solitary existence and Hindu devotees attend in the hope of attaining some spiritual enlightenment. One of the pilgrimage sites is the holy city of Allahabad on the banks of the River Ganges, where devoted Hindus bathe in the river to wash away their sins.

Sacraments and rites of passage

The Sixteen Sacraments (*samskaras*) are acts of purification and refinement for developing body, mind and intellect. They are performed at important stages of life during religious ceremonies involving certain rituals. Today, not all Hindus observe all the *samskaras*, especially in the West, but they may be remembered at other times or incorporated into other ceremonies; for example, the sacred thread ceremony may not be performed at a young age but at the time of marriage.

Garbhadhana is performed after the wedding ceremony for the ability to bear children and for the conferment of a life-giving soul upon the fetus.

Punasavana is performed after the second or third month of pregnancy for the strong physical growth of the unborn child.

Simantonnayana is performed in the sixth or eighth month of pregnancy for the mental wellbeing of the unborn child.

Jatakarma is performed at birth. The newborn child is welcomed into the world by putting a small amount of honey into its mouth and whispering the name of God into its ear.

Namakaran is a naming ceremony performed about 11 days after birth. Names are intended to have meaning and provide inspiration throughout the life of the individual. Names, which may have Sanskrit origins, are often chosen in accordance with the date of birth and associated horoscope, and the scriptures. In some cases, a priest may be asked to help choose a suitable name.

Nishkramana is the ceremony at which the child is introduced to nature at about 4 months of age by being taken outside and exposed to the rays of the sun.

Annaprasana is the time when the baby is weaned at around 6–7 months of age. A special meal is cooked while specific Vedic mantras are chanted. The father feeds the child a few grains of rice before a priest, and prayers are then offered for the wellbeing of the child in the future.

Choodakarma (Mundan) is performed at around the age of 3 years, often in the presence of many family members and friends. During the ceremony all the child's hair is shaved off, both to rid the child of impure thoughts and also to allow the development of the skull to be checked. A further purpose of the ceremony is to symbolize the loosening of ties between a child and its mother as, by the age of 3, breast-feeding has usually ceased. A common misconception is that this *samskara* is equivalent to confirmation or baptism. In the Hindu faith, a child is born a Hindu and no further ceremonies are required.

Karnavedha is the ritual piercing of the ear lobes at 3–5 years of age. This is still popular with girls and has its origins in the scriptures, which state that it prevents disease.

Upanayama (Yajnopaveer or the sacred thread ceremony) takes place when a child reaches school age and is introduced to the teacher or guru and given the sacred thread. The sacred thread consists of three strands, which remind the child of the threefold obligation:

- to promote knowledge gained from all sages, thinkers and scientists
- to respect and care for one's parents and ancestors
- to serve the society and country in which he/she lives.

The ceremony stresses the life of morality and sexual purity that each person is expected to live. The threads are reminders of these vows and it is important that they are not removed except *in extremis.*

Vidyarambha occurs at the beginning of education and is normally performed at school before the first lesson in which pupils learn the meaning of a traditional Hindu prayer aimed at the acquisition of sound intellect.

Samavartana. On finishing education, a graduation sacrament is performed to signify that a person is ready to take part in the social and economic activities of the community.

Vivaha (marriage) marks the start of the second phase of life – that of the householder. Two individuals who are considered to be compatible are joined in a lifelong partnership during a ceremony of many parts, which may take several hours to complete.

Vanaprastha marks the third stage of life, which begins at the age of 50 years, as a person prepares to withdraw from a worldly life in preparation for a spiritual life.

Sanyasa heralds the final stage of life at 75 years of age when all desires and worldly connections with relatives and material goods are renounced. The person becomes a *sanyasi* and traditionally wanders from place to place; householders have a duty to provide them with food and shelter if needed.

Antyeshti (death rites) is the final sacrament performed at death. Hindus believe that the physical body dies while the soul or *atman* lives on. The body is believed to be made of five physical elements: fire, water, earth, air and space. By cremating the body, it is allowed to return to its constituent elements.

Family

Family is extremely important to Hindus and forms the backbone of their society. Traditionally, Hindus live in an extended family where all work for the good of the family even when they get married, and where women join the husband's household following marriage.

Although it is now more common for Hindus in the West to live in more nuclear families, the notion of needing to find children suitable marriage partners is more understandable once the importance of maintaining the family structure is appreciated. Marriages arranged by family elders continue to be common practice and may occur across international boundaries. It can be difficult for a young bride from India to join her new husband's family in the West with the additional problems of adjusting to a different climate, culture and language. The isolation of such a situation may manifest itself in various ways including emotional ill-health.

Women are highly regarded in the Hindu faith and the status of mother is very high ranking; indeed, the concept of mother as a provider is extended to include nature and the earth. Hindu scriptures, such as the *Mahabharata*, state that adoration of one's mother is equal to adoration of God. Respect for elders is also encouraged and it is common for family members and others to bow to parents and elders.

Dress

Although many Hindus in the West wear western clothes, traditional garments are regularly worn by some and on special days by others. Traditional attire for women is the sari, which is a long piece of fabric wound several times around the body and the loose end passed over the left shoulder. It is worn over a petticoat-like garment and a *choli*, which is a tight short blouse which clips up at the front. An alternative is a long smock over trousers; a simpler version of this may also be worn by men.

Many Hindus apply a *tilak* to their foreheads between their eyes before prayers. A *tilak* is a red dot that is applied to the middle of the forehead made from a paste of sandalwood, turmeric or sindoor (zinc oxide) mixed with vermillion powder. Some women wear the tilak using a decorative, self-adhesive fabric. Sandalwood has a pleasant smell and a cooling effect – a reminder that the head should remain calm and cool. Spiritually, the mark serves as a symbol of the third eye of God and the seat of memory, which is believed to be housed in the forehead. Thus, the *tilak* symbolizes retention of the memory of the Lord. Married women often wear a *tilak* or *bindi* as a reminder of their vows and symbol of their marriage, and they cease the practice if they are widowed.

Henna or *mehendi* is a powdered leaf which is made into a paste that can be used to color hair or decorate the skin. It leaves a golden-brown pattern on the skin for several days. It has become common to decorate the hands and feet of a bride for her wedding using elaborate patterns, which may center around a single point designed to see off the 'evil eye'.

Food and drink

Hindus believe that the behavior of all living things is determined by the food that they eat. Thus, many Hindus are strict vegetarians, though some will eat eggs and chicken, and others allow fish or other seafood. Pork is not eaten because the pig is seen as a scavenger and the meat is considered unclean. The strictness of the vegetarian diet varies according to caste and regional traditions.

The lacto-vegetarian diet (fruit, vegetables, pulses, grains, nuts, sugar, honey, milk and milk products) is believed to provide the perfect balance between eating and elimination, and thus maintenance of physical and mental health. All living things are said to possess three qualities in different proportions:

- *sattvic* or purity (milk, fruit, vegetables and grains)
- *rajasic* or activity (meat, alcohol, eggs, spicy foods)
- *tamasic* or inertia (putrefied, over-ripe or rotten).

These qualities will be conferred in the same proportions in which the foods are eaten.

Reverence for the cow probably dates back to early times in India. The cow provided milk and milk products to eat, and its dung was used in house building and for fuel, while the bull was used to plough the fields and was also a means of travel and carrying goods. It is no wonder that to kill a cow was therefore regarded as a sin. The scriptures state that to kill a cow is forbidden and it is even illegal in some Indian states.

Food has religious significance for Hindus in several ways. Preparation of special foods on festival days for communal enjoyment is a way of remembering culture and also sharing with fellow human beings. On these days, as in regular private and public worship, offerings of food are made to the images of God as a way of remembering that food is part of God's creation. Hindu individuals and temples also often arrange for the free distribution of food as part of their duty to society.

Fasting is common on particular days of the week, special holidays and in conjunction with special prayers. In Hindu culture, fasting can vary from complete abstinence to missing one meal per day. The timing and amount of food intake should be considered when providing education about disease processes that may be affected by fasting, such as diabetes and pregnancy (see Chapter 9).

General health issues

Late-onset diabetes, hypertension and other cardiovascular disorders are common in individuals of Indian ethnic origin. Furthermore, control of diabetes and hypertension may be more difficult for Asians used to a traditional high-carbohydrate and high-fat diet. Changes in diet and physical activity following emigration to the West are also thought to contribute to the development of these common chronic diseases.

Many traditional Hindus have a distrust of hospitals, which are perceived to be a place to die when one is extremely ill. Indeed, in South Asia, home births are quite common in order to avoid hospitals. In Western cultures where hospital births are the norm, Hindu immigrants may be exposed to the hospital system for the first time when enrolling for prenatal care. Contact with healthcare professionals during pregnancy and delivery is an excellent opportunity for patient education and encouragement to return on a regular basis for well-woman care.

Traditional Hindus believe in the presence of three body humors: wind (*vata*), bile (*pitta*) and phlegm (*kapha*). As in other Asian cultures, the hot and cold theory applies to foods and its effects on the three humors. Disruption of this equilibrium is believed to cause illness and therefore some foods are preferred over others depending on the illness. Hospital patients may ask family members to bring food from home, because food prepared in the hospital may have come in contact with other forbidden foods. Vomiting and/or incontinence may be viewed as signs of a 'bad death'.

Pain and suffering may be interpreted as retribution for sinful acts/deeds in this or previous lives, which may impact on self-reported pain levels. Patients may demonstrate a reluctance to use pain-relief medications and prefer to use meditation.

Patients may refuse to take medications as capsules, because the gelatin coating may be derived from cows or pigs. Blood transfusion and blood products are generally considered acceptable.

Family elders have a strong influence when making medical decisions and patients will often defer to them for treatment decisions. Men have a responsibility to look after women and will be reluctant to leave any female patient in the presence of an unfamiliar man; a same-sex caregiver or chaperone is preferred, if available. Hindu women may also be quite shy and should be gowned in a manner that protects modesty.

Hindus are meticulous about hygiene and personal cleanliness, because the concept of purity is important to Hindu life. Showers are preferred to baths. It is common practice to remove your shoes before entering a Hindu home to avoid bringing in dirt.

Hindu patients may have specific times for prayer and meditation, which are generally after bathing in the early morning and in the early evening. They may also have a desire to keep religious statues or pictures close by.

Some Hindus will wear protective jewelry or sacred strings at all times. If it is absolutely necessary to remove these objects for surgical procedures, this should be carefully explained and they should be given to relatives for safekeeping.

Contraception and reproduction

Women are considered temporarily impure when menstruating and following childbirth, because bodily secretions are considered unclean. However, there are no specific religious rules or restrictions regarding contraception or pregnancy. While there are generally no specific prohibitions to abortion, it is discouraged but accepted in extenuating circumstances where the wellbeing of mother, unborn child or the family are threatened.

Prayers and ceremonies of purification and wellbeing, which were described earlier in this chapter, are undertaken at various stages of pregnancy and following the birth. 'Hot' yoga (e.g. Bikram yoga) should perhaps be avoided during pregnancy, because of the effects of dehydration on the developing fetus and the increased risk of neural tube defects associated with excessive heat exposure in the first trimester. Other forms of yoga, low-impact exercise and meditation are acceptable during pregnancy.

During pregnancy, women who are true vegans require additional vitamin supplementation, screening for serum vitamin B_{12} levels and possibly injections of vitamin B_{12}. Amniocentesis and prenatal diagnosis are generally acceptable. Prenatal ultrasonography to determine the sex of the fetus can also be a popular practice in Western culture. The birth of a boy is highly prized in that it allows both the family name to continue and avoids the potentially vast expense of having to pay for the wedding of a daughter.

Hindu male infants, unlike Muslims, are not generally circumcised. The Hindu religion does not allow circumcision as it was not described in Sanskrit literature. However, depending on the degree of acculturation, some Hindus in Western countries allow their sons to be circumcised.

Failure to conceive is problematic for some couples and, where assisted conception is unavailable or inaccessible, a man may leave his wife to seek another who may bear him children.

Stillbirth or neonatal death before 7 months' gestation requires no religious ceremony because the soul is not thought to enter the body until this time. The bodies of children and fetuses are generally buried because their personalities are not fully formed and therefore do not need the purification provided through cremation.

Autopsy on a fetus or infant is generally acceptable only if legally necessary.

Breast-feeding. Some women believe colostrum to be impure in some way and are inclined to avoid breast-feeding in the first few days after delivery. Advice and education regarding the benefits of colostrum to the infant may therefore be needed. Women with a South-Asian background commonly mix breast- and bottle-feeding rather than exclusively breast-feed. Although mixed feeding is discouraged by Western breast-feeding advisers, many Asian women undertake it very successfully.

Sexuality

In the Hindu faith, human sexuality has a clear purpose – to foster a beautiful union between man and wife with the aim of procreation. The Hindu wise men have long maintained that sexual attraction between the sexes is normal, and that sexual intercourse is healthy and to be encouraged provided it takes place in an appropriate context. Sex before marriage and adulterous relationships are discouraged.

Sex between members of the same sex cannot create offspring and is regarded as a misuse of a God-given gift. There is currently an increasing number of people infected with HIV and AIDS worldwide, and homosexuality is considered by Hindus to be responsible for a significant number of these cases.

Death

Family members may be reluctant for a diagnosis of terminal illness to be disclosed to a dying relative, because it may be seen as hastening the death by destroying hope. Dying patients may choose to fast to ensure that the body is pure at the time of death.

Autopsies are not generally acceptable to families unless legally necessary, though organ donation can be acceptable. Suicide is strongly condemned because the taking of one's life prematurely results in forces of karma that lead to much more pain and suffering in the reincarnated life than would have been encountered otherwise.

After a person dies, the body is washed and wrapped in white cloth; men are washed and wrapped by men and women by women. The white cloths signify purity and peace. The body may be placed on the ground to signify its return to mother earth. Cremation is generally the funeral rite of choice for adults in Hindu culture and, traditionally, should be carried out within 24 hours of death. Cremation is seen as a means of purifying the dead and expediting the travel of the soul from this world to the next life. Hindu women generally wear white saris during mourning, but may wear red in some parts of India. Traditionally, men wash in cold water at the funeral site and the oldest son, husband or nearest male relative lights the funeral pyre. Prayers for peace are recited and offerings made to the fire. The ashes are collected 3 days later and scattered according to family traditions. Some families return to India in order to scatter the ashes in the River Ganges.

A mourning period of 13 days is traditionally observed after which no further rituals are performed. An exception to this is where families continue to honor their ancestors on the anniversary of their death by making offerings to learned priests and saying prayers.

Clearly, not all of the traditional death rites can be performed in the West and some of the rites take place in the home or in hospital.

Key points – Hinduism

- The Hindu faith is the oldest in the world.
- Women are highly regarded and the status of 'mother' is particularly prized.
- Family elders, especially men, may have a strong influence regarding decision-making, which may extend to healthcare.
- It is common for Hindus to adopt a lactovegetarian diet and to avoid pork or pig products; patients may refuse medication if the capsules are made from gelatin. Fasting is also a common practice.
- Cardiovascular disease and diabetes are common in those of South-Asian origin.
- Many traditional Hindus have a distrust of hospitals; many opt for home births for this reason.

Followers of Islam are called Muslims. There are estimated to be more than 1.3 billion Muslims worldwide accounting for about one-fifth of the world's population. Indonesia has the largest Muslim community of 200 million people. Approximately one-third of the world's Muslims live in non-Muslim states; India has the largest Muslim

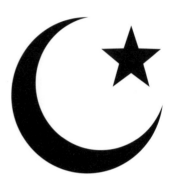

minority of 120 million people, while China has at least 60 million Muslims. There are about 1.6 million Muslims in the UK and 6 million in the USA. The crescent moon has become the accepted symbol of Islam.

Islam means peace and submission to God. The term Muslims was first said to have been used by the prophet Abraham. Although the prophet Muhammad is central to the faith, to refer to Muslims as Muhammadans may be viewed as an insult. Followers believe in the divinity of the message of Islam, which is centered around the concept of the one, omnipotent, omniscient God – Allah. The belief in one God and his final messenger, the Prophet Muhammad, is the foundation of Islam. Muslims believe that each prophet, including Jesus, Moses, Noah and Abraham, preached essentially the same message of belief and obedience to one God.

Muhammad's name is not mentioned or heard by a devout Muslim without repetition of the words 'peace be upon him' or another form of similar words; it is also sometimes abbreviated in the written form when the name of Muhammad is mentioned (e.g. PBUH). Love of the Prophet serves as the basis on which devout Muslims try to emulate 'the way of Muhammad' or *sunnah* in all aspects of their daily lives. For example, the Prophet sat on the floor in the belief that this reduced the emotional distance between human beings, ate with his right hand and believed in an uncluttered lifestyle among other things. This is sometimes interpreted and reflected in the ascetic furnishing of a traditional Muslim home and use of the floor for both sitting at home and praying.

Mecca lies in what is now Saudi Arabia and is the most holy place for Muslims. It was the place of Muhammad's birth and final sermon. Muhammad's first revelation was received in Mecca when he was 40 years old. The nature of the revelation at that time challenged Meccan society's theology as well as economic and social injustices. As a result, Meccan tribal chiefs persecuted and tortured many Muslims. In 622 CE, 13 years after the revelation, Muhammad migrated with his followers to Medina, approximately 200 miles north of Mecca. In Medina, Muslims built the first mosque and established the first Islamic state. Medina's society is thought to be the model community for Muslims. Muslims were initially taught to pray towards Jerusalem, but were then ordered by God to pray towards Mecca, where Abraham built the first house of worship. In the year 629 CE, Muhammad marched into Mecca with an increased following in a bloodless liberation of the Meccan tribal system. Mecca remains at the heart of Islam today, as do emulations of the events and rituals as undertaken by Muhammad. Muhammad died in Medina in 632 CE at the age of 63 years.

Sects

The great cultural and historic differences between Muslims from different parts of the world has led to wide variations in the practice of certain rituals and customs. The way Muslims from different cultures deal with disease and interact with healthcare professionals may also vary. However, they all have common ground based on shared theological tenets and moral values.

Sunni and Shia Islam are the two primary sects of the Islamic faith that developed following the death of the prophet Muhammad. The Sunnis believed that the Islamic leader to follow Muhammad should be an elected official known as a caliph. The Shias believed that Muhammad's son-in-law should be the leader, because he did not have a son of his own for a bloodline. This dispute has led to several generations of sectarian strife, though both follow the original teachings of the prophet Muhammad.

Five Pillars of Islam

The Five Pillars of Islam are the five obligations that every Muslim must satisfy in order to lead a good and responsible life. They are:

- Belief (*Shahadah*)
- Prayer (*Salat*)
- Giving alms for the poor (*zakat*)
- Fasting during the month of Ramadan (*sawm*)
- Pilgrimage to Mecca (*Hajj*).

Belief. The conviction that God is the supreme being and Muhammad is His messenger underpins all other beliefs. God is viewed as the creator of the universe, in which all of creation is dependent on him. For instance, both sickness and health occurs with His decree and medication functions only with His sustenance.

Prayers may be offered at any time, but every Muslim should pray with sincerity five times daily as ordered by Muhammad. Muhammad compared the required prayers and purifying of the soul five times a day to washing oneself in a running stream outside one's house five times a day and not leaving a blemish on one's heart. The appointed times for the prayers are between first light and dawn, noon until mid-afternoon, mid-afternoon until sunset, just after sunset and from the time when it is completely dark until midnight or until the next day. Devout Muslims pray towards Mecca.

Giving alms for the poor consists of one-fortieth or 2.5% of one's liquid assets. This money may be given to charities for the poor or may be given to support local Muslim communities. In Muslim countries, the money is collected by the government, but in non-Muslim countries, mosques and charitable institutions organize donations.

Fasting, which includes sexual abstinence, from sunrise to sunset during Ramadan, the ninth month of the Muslim year, is the fourth pillar of Islam. The Muslim calendar is a lunar one and therefore recedes relative to the solar calendar by 11 days each year.

Pilgrimage is the final pillar of Islam. Every observant Muslim is obliged to make a journey to Mecca (*Hajj*) at least once in a lifetime.

Scripture

The Qur'an (Koran) is the holy book of Muslims and represents the words of Allah, conveyed by the angel Gabriel and received by Muhammad. The Qur'an is not a chronological text nor is it a linear story about ancient peoples, but rather a series of chapters and verses. The various parts of the Qur'an were revealed over a period of years to Muhammad and the archangel Gabriel determined where they should be placed. Recitation of the Qur'an is encouraged from a young age and many Muslims can recite the Qur'an in its entirety. Contained within the Qur'an are verses pertaining to social and economic codes by which Muslims should live their lives, as well as verses devoted to the virtues of reason and the glory of God. The interpretation of the guidance within the Qur'an varies between communities; for example, the Qur'an tells Muslims to be modest but dress codes vary widely between communities.

Worship

Islam encourages direct relationships with God and the belief that God will respond in a generous and gracious fashion to the prayers of His people. Therefore no hierarchy of priests, bishops or their equivalent exists in Islam, and there are no sacraments to administer. Prayers in mosques are led by Imams, who can be any male member of the congregation able to recite the Qur'an and deliver a sermon before the congregation during weekly Friday noon prayers. In some communities, an Imam may also undertake a pastoral role such as visiting patients in hospitals. However, some Muslims may prefer to be visited by revered, devout family members or elders of the community whose prayers are regarded as especially worthy.

Hajj

Dhul Hijjah is the most important month in the Muslim calendar. Although a pilgrimage or *Hajj* to Mecca can be undertaken at any time, it does not have the same value as that made at during *Dhul Hijjah*.

Each year, during a 5-day period between the 8th and 13th day of the last month of the Islamic calendar, around 2.5–3 million pilgrims undertake the journey to Mecca and numbers continue to increase annually. The *Hajj* is the culmination of many years of faith and constitutes a very special journey both physically and spiritually.

Since the *Hajj* takes place in a very hot climate and the density of people is enormous, it can have many implications for health, especially for the elderly or those whose health is already compromised. Any pilgrims on long-term medications should be advised to ensure that they have adequate supplies, as medicines may be difficult to access while on pilgrimage. Where possible, prospective pilgrims should also be advised of measures to overcome commonly encountered problems.

Climate. Dehydration is a common problem and occurs quickly in such a hot climate. Pilgrims should be advised to drink plenty of fluid throughout the day, carry water with them and to increase their salt intake or use rehydration salts.

Heat-stroke is another hazard, particularly for men who are prohibited from covering their heads during the pilgrimage. A person with heat-stroke will feel hot to the touch and will not be sweating. Urgent medical attention is needed but, in the meantime, the person should be moved to a cool, shaded place and have their bodies cooled by removing clothes, tepid sponging and fanning.

Sunburn is also a significant risk, especially for the paler skinned. Use of adequate amounts of high-factor sunscreen should be encouraged. An umbrella, particularly a white or pale colored one to reflect the sun, can also be extremely useful.

Vaccination and prophylaxis. The Saudi government made vaccination against meningitis mandatory following the outbreak in British Muslims returning from pilgrimage in 1987.

It is also advisable to be vaccinated against hepatitis A and B due to the potential risks of shaving. Although it is acceptable to have the hair or beard trimmed at the end of the *Hajj*, most men opt for shaving. However, it is not uncommon for the same razor to be used several times on different men, which presents obvious risks of bloodborne diseases, such as hepatitis and HIV. Pilgrims should be made aware of this possibility so that they can insist on a new blade being used.

It is also advisable to ensure that immunity to tetanus, diphtheria and polio are up to date, and protection against typhoid is considered. The proposed itinerary should be checked as some pilgrims may be traveling to other countries after the *Hajj* and may require additional protective measures, such as other vaccinations or antimalarial tablets.

Environment. Patients with diabetes need to be careful about foot care, especially if they have a neuropathy. Removal of footwear for parts of the *Hajj* may result in a person having to walk on hot ground to reclaim their shoes. While this may cause some damage to the healthy foot, a person with a neuropathy may suffer far greater damage because they do not realize that it is happening.

The hot and dusty environment may be very unpleasant for wearers of contact lenses. They should be advised to use lubricating eye drops or to change to spectacles for this period.

Menstruation. Women who are menstruating are ritually unclean and therefore unable to take part in the *Hajj*. A woman may therefore consult her family physician, gynecologist or family planning clinic to try and avoid menstruation when the *Hajj* is approaching. This can be achieved by use of the combined oral contraceptive pill taken continuously for the duration of the trip if appropriate and safe, or by the use of progestogens taken continuously in a dose sufficient to prevent bleeding.

Ramadan

The holy month of Ramadan, the ninth month of the Muslim calendar, is a time for prayer and spiritual purification involving abstinence. As well as abstaining from all food and drink, smoking and sex are also prohibited from dawn until dusk. Conversely, overeating during the hours of darkness is discouraged as this goes against the spirit of Ramadan, which encourages moderation and self-discipline.

Children, pregnant women, the elderly, people who are sick and those traveling are exempt from fasting. However, despite being eligible for exemption or permitted to make up the time at some other point, many people still choose to fast with everyone because of the great spiritual significance Ramadan carries. Most patients can safely fast, but some will benefit from advice and a change in medication schedules or routes of administration (see Chapter 9).

It may be difficult for patients to discuss fasting with their doctor, because they fear that the safety aspect will be overplayed or their doctor will not understand the importance of the fast and therefore not suggest alternative, acceptable treatment. It is not uncommon, therefore, for patients to alter their own regimens sometimes with dangerous consequences (e.g. those with diabetes or epilepsy). Understanding what is permitted and the commitment that many patients have to Ramadan will help healthcare workers to establish a rapport with their Muslim patients and thus avoid some of the pitfalls.

Rites of passage

Although not compulsory in Islam, circumcision is considered an important ritual aimed at improving cleanliness and it is seen as a sign of belonging to the faith. There is no fixed age at which circumcision is performed; it may be undertaken at any time from 7 days after birth to puberty. Circumcisions may be undertaken in a public hospital, in the private sector or in the community by non-professionals. Not surprisingly, complication rates of circumcisions done by non-professionals tend to be higher than those undertaken in hospital, but it is possible that the lack of provision of free services in the public sector may contribute to this. Circumcision should be avoided in the presence of jaundice because of the increased risk of bleeding and genital malformation, such as hypospadias.

In some Muslim cultures, on the seventh day after birth, the baby's hair is shaved off and a gift of its weight in gold or silver is traditionally given to the poor. This is an act that acknowledges the state of purity in which a new baby is born. A sheep is also slaughtered in thanksgiving, and the meat shared among family and the poor. This may, however, be done in a family's home country where the need for food may be greater and enable the extended family to share in the celebration. Alternatively, in the UK and the USA, meat may be ordered from the butcher and distributed locally among friends, family, neighbors and the poor.

The age of consent has been established by Islamic law to be 16 years of age or younger, depending on physiological maturation, which is defined as the first nocturnal emission for boys and menarche for girls.

Family

The family is highly regarded in Muslim culture as the backbone of society. Traditionally, the extended family is the norm, with all the different generations living under one roof. While this affords a greater degree of support in many respects than a nuclear family, the latter may be seen to offer greater personal freedom, especially by second-generation settlers in Western countries.

The man is the head of the family and, whether or not his wife is earning, the man bears the economic responsibility for maintaining the family. Therefore, if he is unemployed or his wife earns more than he does, it can cause problems.

Marriage within Islamic society is strongly encouraged and viewed as the union of both two people as well as two families. According to Islamic thinking, children have the right to be conceived and raised in a secure and loving environment. The undertaking to 'Know your genealogy and respect your blood ties' has been interpreted as children having a right to be born through a valid marriage. A marriage that has been 'arranged' should have the consent and blessing of the individual partners before it proceeds.

Following marriage, the woman traditionally goes to live in the family home of her husband. If this involves leaving her home and her extended family to move to a foreign country, adjustment to culture and society can result in significant psychological morbidity. Furthermore, language problems and feelings of relative social isolation may deter these women from seeking healthcare services.

The parent–child relationship is considered the most important of all human relationships. Therefore, any form of child abuse is considered abhorrent under Islamic law, but this is weighed against the need to discipline a child for the good of society, which may include physical punishment.

Dress

Observant Muslims dress modestly, though the precise interpretation varies depending on the patient's background. The Qur'an states that clothing should not reveal the form of the body and that it should not be light or transparent. This applies to both men and women. Many Muslim women will cover their heads: some will wear a head scarf (hijab), others will wear a loose fine shawl (shayla) and some a face veil with either a slit for their eyes or a fabric mesh across their eyes (chadri). Some Muslim women wear large dark cloaks that cover their entire bodies from head to toe called burqas (covering the entire face) or chadors (which do not cover the face) so that their entire bodies are concealed from the public. Some men will also cover their heads with varying forms of headwear depending on the culture and the community to which they belong.

Although Muslim patients will, at times, have to undress, preservation of modesty where possible will always be appreciated, as with most patients. Even if patients are due for surgery, use of a disposable hat such as the ones used by operating theatre staff provides a means of covering the head without compromising care.

Food and drink

Food eaten by Muslims should be clean and wholesome. The Qur'an prescribes which foods are acceptable and which are forbidden (*haram*). Meat from an animal that has been killed in an unknown way or has died rather than been slaughtered is forbidden. Meat which still contains blood is also unacceptable. Pork and pork products are forbidden, even for medical purposes. However, in exceptional circumstances, if the only food available is forbidden, a Muslim is obliged to eat the food that is generally forbidden in order to preserve his/her life.

Halal food is food that has been prepared according to Islamic law. *Halal* meat comes from animals that have had their throats cut with a knife and all blood drained from them. The knife should be as sharp as possible to bring about death as quickly and painlessly as is feasible, and a prayer is recited during the process. Slaughtering of an animal may not be performed in front of another animal. Most hospital and community meal providers now provide *halal* food.

Alcohol is strictly forbidden in Islam in line with the general principles of maintaining the health of the body and mind. As an intoxicant that clouds the mind, it may upset the harmony of an individual with their community and environment.

Medicine derived from forbidden food is unacceptable. Anything which has a gelatin capsule (e.g. antibiotic or analgesic capsules), is gelatin-derived (e.g. some plasma expanders) or is otherwise derived from pigs (e.g. porcine insulin) should be replaced with an acceptable alternative whenever possible. Similarly, medicine that is alcohol based is not allowed.

General health issues

Islam maintains a positive view of the body and obliges Muslims to keep their bodies in a state of health as much as they are able. This is partly expressed by the physical movements including bowing, kneeling and prostration involved in praying, which are designed to blend the spiritual with the physical. However, any activity that will jeopardize health or worsen an existing condition is discouraged. For this reason, those who are physically frail are exempted from praying in this way. For instance, if a patient is bedridden, movements may be minimized by simulating the motions of prayer by nodding of the head or, if that is not possible, by moving the eyes. This is important, because many Muslims feel inadequate if they do not complete their prayers.

Prayers may also be a source of spiritual support especially during the time of illness. Spirituality is also thought to play a role in physical health; illness, particularly emotional and mental disorders, is sometimes ascribed to a lack of faith.

Views on medical treatment are culturally as well as theologically influenced. Some Muslims cite the Prophet's teachings such as 'God has provided a cure for every disease' and 'Seek medical treatment', while others turn to the great Islamic scholar of the 9th century, Ahmad Ibn Hanbal, who said, 'Medication is permissible, but abandonment of it is preferable'. Therefore, while some Muslims believe taking medication is a religious duty in that it preserves health, others believe it is preferable to avoid treatment.

Islamic culture also directly influences the doctor–patient relationship. For instance, the association of unrelated men and women is discouraged and physical contact is strictly prohibited; this means that the usual social pleasantries such as shaking hands may be inappropriate.

While an exception is made in Islamic law for the doctor–patient relationship, it is still common for women to wish to be attended exclusively by women, especially if examination of the genitalia is required. Likewise, if an interpreter is required, some patients may feel more relaxed if a same-sex interpreter can be found. However, if no female physician is available, most Muslim women will accept care from a male attendant at least in an emergency.

Hygiene. Although the Prophet lived in a harsh desert climate where water was scarce, he insisted his followers maintain good hygiene. However, cleansing rituals that might adversely affect health are strongly discouraged as an act of misplaced piety.

Prayers are offered in a clean place, usually on a prayer carpet, directed towards Mecca. Before praying, a cleansing ritual is performed, which involves passing clean water over the mouth, nostrils, hands, face and forearms, washing the feet, and wiping the head and ears.

After using the lavatory, the anus and genitals should be washed with clean water. In Muslim countries, this need is usually met by having a shower hose next to the toilet or a bidet in a private bathroom. Provision of a jug or other receptacle and water container or tap nearby from which the jug may be filled is a substitute, which any home or institution visited by devout Muslims can accommodate.

Another cleansing ritual involves rinsing of the entire body after sexual intercourse, ejaculation and, for women, after menstruation has ceased each month.

Contraception and reproduction

As with other religions, there are a variety of views about the use of contraception. On the one hand, there are those who strictly ban contraception and, on the other, there are those who are concerned with global population control and encourage strategic family planning. In practice, most Muslims fall somewhere between the two extremes and family sizes are reducing, especially in developed countries.

Certain methods of contraception, such as the intrauterine system containing levonorgestrel or other progestogen-based methods that may cause irregular bleeding, may be less appealing to some women than those associated with predictable bleeding. For other women, the use of intrauterine contraceptive devices with the attendant reduction in need for future medical consultations, especially if it might involve being seen by a male doctor, outweighs the potential disadvantages of bleeding problems.

Non-menstrual bleeding (e.g. after a Pap/Papanicolau/cervical)smear or other gynecologic procedure) may be mistaken for menstruation and may make women reluctant to have their intrauterine device checked or have smear tests. If healthcare professionals are aware of this and can advise appropriately, the uptake rate of these valuable checks could be increased.

Infertility. Children are considered to have a right to know their parentage fully. Therefore, for observant Muslims, in-vitro fertilization and artificial insemination can only occur with sperm from the woman's spouse. Adoption and surrogate motherhood are also frowned on due to the uncertainty of parentage.

Abortion. In general, Islam discourages the termination of pregnancy. Some Islamic scholars, however, refer to the Prophet's teaching that the introduction of the soul into the body does not occur until the 120th day of life (17 weeks from conception or 19 weeks from the first day of the last menstrual period). They thus defend the right to abortion before 120 days after conception. First trimester chorionic villus sampling or first trimester nuchal translucency testing may therefore be more acceptable, because a termination for an anomaly could still be performed before the ensoulment of the fetus.

Genetic testing. Marriage between relatives is common in Muslim communities of South Asian and Arab origin; in the UK, as many as 50% of couples of Pakistani origin are married to first cousins. In social terms, the advantages are that each family is well known to the other, and any material and financial assets are kept within the extended family. Unfortunately, the practice has also led to high levels of consanguinity and an increasing number of children with otherwise rare autosomal disorders born to Muslim parents. Thus, there is clearly a need for accessible genetic counseling in this population. While some couples would choose to continue a pregnancy knowing that there is no chance that their baby will survive, others may choose to terminate a pregnancy after careful consideration.

Birth. Within minutes of birth, a devout father will take his newborn infant in his arms and whisper the declaration of faith – 'There is no God but Allah and Muhammad is his messenger' – into the baby's right ear. This is both an affirmation of the central tenet of Islam and also a symbol of the responsibilities of the father in his child's upbringing. Ideally, peace and privacy should be afforded for this to be done.

In some Muslim cultures, a respected elder of the family may rub softened date onto the tongue or palate of the newborn in the hope that he or she will grow up to be sweet in temperament and may inherit some of the good qualities of that relative.

It is common, especially among Muslims from the Indian subcontinent, to tie a small pouch containing a prayer to the infants neck or wrist with black string (*taweez*). It is thought to protect the infant from ill health and should only be removed if strictly necessary.

Breast-feeding. Religious teaching encourages breast-feeding until 2 years of age. However, the imperative for modesty prohibits a woman revealing her breasts to anyone other than her husband, other women and immediate family, and the lack of privacy in an average postnatal ward may produce a conflict of interest. Babies may be breast-fed by another Muslim woman, but the children must be informed when they are older, as any children fed by the same woman are classed as siblings and may therefore not marry each other according to Muslim law.

Women of Bangladeshi origin believe that colostrum is harmful to the baby, and substitute honey and water or formula for the first few days of life. This belief is not based on religious teaching and reshaping of views would be clearly beneficial for the health of these newborn babies.

Sexuality

While the Prophet encouraged his followers to have a healthy sexual relationship based on love, intimacy and respect, today's social circumstances have stigmatized sexual intercourse. The Prophet taught that men should please their wives both emotionally and sexually, but today many Muslims are taught that sex is only for the purpose of procreation and for women to please men.

Many women from traditional cultures are unaware of what sexual intercourse entails until marriage. For this reason, many couples, especially women, will suffer from low sexual desire, orgasmic dysfunction and vaginismus. Men may suffer with erectile and ejaculatory disorders, and because of the stigma (sometimes ignorance) associated with sexual dysfunction, these problems often present later as general marital difficulties.

Sexual intercourse outside marriage and between homosexuals is forbidden according to Islamic law. Anal intercourse and vaginal intercourse during menstruation are also forbidden. While having homosexual inclinations is not considered a sin, homosexual sex is.

Death

Since Muslims believe in the hereafter, death marks a transition from one life to the next. A dying person will repeat their belief in Allah (*Shahadah*), while their assembled family recite prayers. Praying with a dying person and being responsible for their body after death is a great honor. It is customary for a dying person to be visited by many friends and family, and preferably to die at home. A Muslim will also wish to die facing Mecca. In hospital, lifting the usual restrictions of no more than two visitors and turning the bed towards Mecca may be much appreciated.

After death, the body is washed three times and wrapped in unstitched pieces of white cloth. It is then carried to the place of burial and preferably laid on its right side directly on the soil with the face towards Mecca. Burial takes place as soon after death as possible: 'The sun should not be allowed to set twice on a dead body' is an expression meaning that it should be buried within 24 hours. Following prayers, members of the community and sometimes family bury the body. In predominantly Muslim countries, it is possible to bury a dead person within a matter of hours. In the UK and other non-Muslim-dominated countries, it can be more difficult though the provision of services is improving. In order to bury the dead quickly, there should be no unnecessary delay in issuing the death certificate and releasing the body if the death occurs in hospital.

Autopsy will delay the burial and may cause great consternation to the family, particularly as some believe that the dead body may feel pain. If the autopsy is to obtain further information about the cause of death without a clear medicolegal need, it must be made clear to the family that they are under no obligation to agree to it. Given the high prevalence of consanguinity, it may be helpful to evaluate stillborn fetuses by X-ray if autopsy is not permissible.

The duration and expression of mourning is culturally determined. It often lasts for 3 days and, during this time, many friends and family may visit the home of the deceased to say prayers and remember the life of the deceased. The period of official mourning may last around 3–4 months for a widow, by which time it will be clear if she is carrying the child of the deceased. If she is pregnant, the period of mourning ends with the delivery of the child irrespective of the time since her husband died. During this time she is likely to remain in the family home, but religious dispensation does allow her to travel to seek medical advice and care.

Since Muslims believe that the body is entrusted to God and life is given and taken away by Him, suicide and euthanasia are forbidden. Withdrawal of life support is also a contentious decision. Organ donation may also be controversial, because the body and its organs are not believed to belong to the deceased. However, some Muslims believe that, if a donated organ will save a life, transplantation is permitted under Islamic doctrine, which holds that 'necessity permits the prohibited'.

Key points – Islam

- Muslims believe in one God (Allah), that all is determined by God and that his final messenger on earth was the Prophet Muhammad.
- The codes for living are known as the 'Five Pillars of Islam', which involve declaring one's faith, praying five times daily, fasting during Ramadan, giving money to the poor and making a pilgrimage to Mecca (*Hajj*) at least once in a lifetime.
- Those planning a pilgrimage should be advised of the potential for dehydration, heat stroke and sunburn in hot climates and educated about preventative measures. Up-to-date vaccination against tetanus, diphtheria and polio, as well as meningitis and hepatitis A and B, is also advisable.
- Muslims avoid pork and porcine derivatives and non-pork meat must be produced in a particular way (*halal*). Medicine derived from forbidden food is unacceptable.
- Islamic culture may affect the doctor–patient relationship; women may prefer to be treated by a female physician.

There are over 14 million Jews worldwide comprising 0.23% of the world's population. Approximately 7 million Jews live in the USA, 5 million in Israel and another 2 million throughout the rest of the world. Today, the degree to which Jews adhere to religious observance varies, or they may differ in opinion as to the expression of religious beliefs; however, there is a strong cultural element to being Jewish – food, festivals and ritual – which is shared and widely practiced.

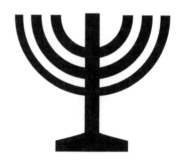

The Jewish faith is around 4000 years old. Jews believe that they are God's chosen people and part of a greater divine purpose. The Jewish faith began with Abraham being called by God to settle in the land of Canaan. Abraham's grandson Jacob was promised many sons and had 12. The tribes of Israel were named after the sons and the most powerful was Judah from which the name 'Jew' is derived.

During a period of slavery to the Egyptians, God spoke to Moses from a burning bush, which was not being consumed by the fire. God told Moses to go to Pharoah and demand that the Israelites be set free. After 10 plagues visited on the Egyptians by God, the Israelites were freed and Moses led the exodus from Egypt. They traveled for 40 years until they reached the Promised Land of Canaan (later known as Palestine). During the Exodus, God gave Moses the Ten Commandments and a series of other laws by which they were to live. These laws are still observed today by Orthodox Jews.

When settled in Canaan, the Israelites appointed a series of judges including Samuel and Gideon to rule over them before they then had a series of kings. The first King, Saul, was succeeded by David and then David's son Solomon. David wrote many of the psalms in the Jewish bible and was greatly loved. Solomon built the Temple in Jerusalem, which was fabled for its beauty. The Menorah, the seven-branched candlestick, is an ancient Jewish symbol representing the candlestick that stood in this Temple. The Temple was destroyed and rebuilt twice. The most extensive rebuilding was by Herod the Great, but the project had barely been completed, long after Herod's death, when the Romans destroyed it. It was never rebuilt after this and the Western Wall is all that remains. As a consequence, emphasis moved away from animal sacrifice in the Temple to worshipping in the synagogue, with rabbis safeguarding the Jewish traditions, and the religion has remained this way ever since.

The Jews have had internal divisions since the times of the Pharisees and Sadducees. There are still divisions today with each offering what they believe to be the 'true version' of the faith. There are four main groups: Orthodox, Reform, Conservative and Reconstructionist. The latter three groups form the Progressive or Liberal movement.

Ultra-Orthodox Jews live in tight-knit communities and are known as the *hassidim* or pious ones. They originated in Eastern Europe, particularly Poland, but there are groups in the UK, USA and Israel, as well as elsewhere. Yiddish is spoken within the community and there is little contact with people outside this group.

Scripture

The Jewish bible is central to the faith. It is written in Hebrew and contains 39 books as in the Christian Old Testament, but the books are in a different order. The Jewish bible is called the *TeNaKh* and comprises three parts: the Torah or Law, *Nev'im* or Prophets and *Ketuvim* or Writings. The Torah, together with the Sabbath, are celebrated as God's greatest gifts to the Jewish people.

The Torah consists of the five books of Moses: Genesis, Exodus, Leviticus, Numbers and Deuteronomy. Reading aloud passages from the Torah is an important part of Jewish worship and to be asked to do so is a very great honor. In the Orthodox community, reading from the Torah in this way is only open to men. Passages from the Torah are read in the synagogue on the Sabbath, festival mornings, and on Monday and Thursday mornings.

Prescribed selections from the Prophets, which contains eight books, are read in synagogues on the Sabbath, festivals and fasting days.

The third section of the bible contains writings and includes the Psalms. Although it is regarded as less important than the other sections, the Psalms are regularly used in synagogue worship, and readings from this section are used on festival days.

Worship

Much of Jewish tradition and faith is expressed in the home, which is regarded as the main focal point for a religious Jewish life. The synagogue is the Jewish holy place for public worship.

The Sabbath or *Shabbat* is a day of rest and relaxation, and is enshrined in the Ten Commandments. It recalls the fact that, according to the Torah, God made the world in 6 days and on the 7th day he rested. Jewish scriptures give strong reasons as to why Jews should observe and zealously guard the Sabbath. First, the idea that rest from work is a creative act of God and, secondly, that following the Jewish exodus, God instigated the Sabbath so that all people and animals should have at least 1 day a week when they did not work.

Shabbat begins at sunset on Friday and ends at sunset on Saturday. As sunset varies throughout the year, it will be mid-afternoon in the winter and quite late in the evening in the summer months in the western hemisphere. Orthodox Jews adhere to the exact times of sunset and will expect their children to finish school early during the winter and for adults to finish any form of work early on a Friday afternoon. Progressive Jews vary in their interpretation of the beginning of *Shabbat* with some choosing to commence early in the summer months at around 8 PM and others using 6 PM as a guide throughout the year.

The Sabbath provides time to study the Torah, visit the synagogue for public worship and prayer, and spend time with family and friends. Traditional Jewish law bans any form of work on this day and Orthodox Jews interpret this to mean carrying out any form of business, using any form of transport, doing shopping or housework, switching equipment on and off, spending money, and using electricity and the telephone. Some followers interpret the laws to prohibit signing hospital consent forms for medical procedures that occur on the Sabbath, pressing elevator buttons, or ringing call-buttons or doorbells in the hospital setting. (Culturally sensitive hospitals in the USA have activated special *Shabbat* elevators in high-rise hospitals that stop automatically on every floor from sundown on Fridays to sundown on Saturdays.) In Orthodox communities in both the USA and UK, the faithful may mark the neighborhood with wire lines attached to electric posts that can be considered 'home' territory to allow their followers more freedom of movement during the *Shabbat*.

The Sabbath begins with the lighting of two or more candles by the mother and children of the Jewish household. The mother then offers a prayer for the well-being of her husband and family. This is then followed by a blessing for the family by the father. Afterwards, the family have a meal, which is followed by singing traditional songs and saying grace.

Home. The Jewish home is considered to be a sacred place and is central to the maintenance of Jewish faith and culture. It will often be marked by a *mezuzah*, which is a small parchment scroll within a container attached to the upper third of all door posts, except for those leading to the bathroom, toilet and garage. The scroll contains verses from Deuteronomy (the *Shema*). The *mezuzah* is a requirement of the Torah and Orthodox Jews will kiss their fingertips before reaching to touch it as a mark of respect for God and the Torah.

Jewish tradition places strong emphasis on the provision of food and hospitality for family, friends and strangers, especially those who are in the middle or at the end of a long journey. It is considered an act of great kindness or '*mitzvah*' to provide a meal and hospitality for those who would not otherwise be able to celebrate the holy day properly.

Prayer is the most important spiritual activity for a Jew. It is regarded as a duty or '*mitzvah*' and represents commitment to the covenant that God made with their ancestors. Traditional synagogues hold three services a day: morning, afternoon and evening. In Orthodox synagogues, a minimum of 10 men must be present before prayers can be offered. This rule does not apply in Reform and Progressive synagogues. Reciting of prayers may be marked by a rocking motion as the religious verses are recited.

Symbols of prayer. There are various symbols of prayer worn by Jews. The *tallit* or prayer shawl is a garment with fringes at its four corners in accordance with the bible and is worn by men, draped across their backs at morning prayer only. *Terfillin* or phylacteries are small cube-shaped leather boxes containing four passages from the scriptures that are attached to the forehead and left arm by long, winding straps. These are also worn during morning prayer, but not on the Sabbath or festival days. Both *terfillin* and *tallit* may be worn by women in Progressive synagogues, but not in Orthodox circles. The *yarmulke* or skullcap is worn by Jewish men. It is believed that praying bareheaded is greatly disrespectful to God. Jews who observe religious laws more zealously will wear the *yarmulke* at all times, but most Jewish men wear it only when praying or en route to and from the synagogue. Young Orthodox American boys may also wear *yarmulkes* embroidered with popular cartoon characters to ensure compliance with covering their heads, while simultaneously deferring to popular culture.

Religious roles. In the Orthodox community, women sit separately from the men in the synagogue and are not permitted to officiate in any way. Within the Progressive movement, the ways in which families and congregations interpret Jewish law are very diverse; women and men may sit in mixed pews in the synagogue, and women may become cantors or be ordained as rabbis.

Originally, the rabbi was solely responsible for teaching the Torah, and interpreting Jewish law and rabbinical writings. Today, devoted followers will still turn to their rabbis to make decisions large and small, including decisions over medical care (e.g. a worshipper may seek the rabbi's approval for a medically indicated hysterectomy for a cancer of the uterus). Over the last 200 years, however, rabbis have taken on a pastoral role as well, in much the same way as Christian ministers. They may visit the sick in hospital, visit the homes of people who are lonely or unwell, and officiate at synagogues.

Festivals

There are many Jewish festivals and holy days throughout the year, but it is important to differentiate holy holidays (the 'high holy days') that have religious significance from the many festivals that are celebrated as a tradition. The exact dates vary from year to year as they are based on a lunar calendar. During the 'high holy days', Orthodox Jews may be seen wearing white canvas shoes (no leather or animal products) to symbolize their humility.

Rosh Hashanah or Jewish New Year has solemn overtones as it is a time of self-examination and remembrance of past deeds and faults, and there are long services in the synagogue. At home, Sabbath eve is marked with a meal during which a piece of bread or apple is dipped into honey; this represents the produce of the land (bread or apple) and the hoped for sweetness of the year to come (honey).

Yom Kippur is the Day of Atonement and takes place 9 days after Rosh Hashanah. This is the most holy and solemn day in the Jewish calendar when Jews ask God for his forgiveness. The days between Rosh Hashanah and Yom Kippur are regarded as an opportunity to put right wrongdoings and ask forgiveness from friends, family and neighbors for any wrong deeds. It is also believed that one cannot ask God's forgiveness for oneself unless one has forgiven others first.

Sukkot. The festival of Sukkot or tabernacles begins a few days after Yom Kippur. The festival recalls the goodness of God in creation and is a reminder that nothing in the world is permanent. During Sukkot, Jews may build tabernacles in their homes and synagogues that are open to the sky. Traditionally, people lived and slept in the tabernacles for the duration of the festival (8 days), but it is more usual, especially in Western countries, to have a communal and symbolic tabernacle at the synagogue. In Orthodox neighborhoods in New York City, many Jewish families build their own temporary Sukkot huts and celebrate with picnics in the huts for the duration of the festival until the structure is taken down to be stored until the following year.

Sukkot ends with Simchat Torah, which is really another festival in its own right. During this festival, the Torah is read by men, women and children (except in Orthodox synagogues) and 'bridegrooms' are elected from the community as a reminder that all Jews are 'married' to the Torah. The festivals of Sukkot and Simchat Torah end and begin cycles of reading from the Torah, respectively.

Hannukah. The festival of lights or Hannukah (Chanukah) is celebrated over 8 days in December and is not a religious festival, but a recollection of an unlikely military victory during the 2nd century BCE. Hannukah recalls the miracle of how the *menorah* (seven-branched candlestick) remained alight in the Temple for 8 days even though it only had enough oil for 1 day. This minor holiday has been timed closely to coincide with the Western Christmas holidays in which Jewish children receive 8 days of Hannukah gifts, sing traditional holiday songs, eat chocolate candy wrapped with gold foil in the shape of money ('gelt') and play the traditional game of the dreidel (a children's spinning top).

Purim. The late winter/early spring festival of Purim celebrates the story of Esther and her cousin Mordechai in the book of Esther. Esther, a Jewish queen, foiled attempts by the evil Haman to destroy the entire Jewish people. During this festival, parts of the book of Esther are read in the synagogue. In the USA, this festival has been adapted to resemble the American celebration of Halloween. During Purim, children dress up in colorful costumes representing 'good queen' Esther and the other characters of the story and eat shortbread cookies filled with fruit jellies called Hamantaschen, which are shaped like the tri-cornered hat supposedly worn by Haman. As a part of the Purim celebration, the children also make 'graggers', which are noisemakers.

Passover or *Pesach* celebrates the exodus of the Jews from slavery in Egypt. It lasts for 8 days for Jews outside Israel, but 7 days for those in

Israel. This is another holy holiday, but happens to coincide closely with the Christian celebration of Easter.

Passover is regarded as a celebration of the power of God and is also a reminder of the covenant made by God with Abraham. Passover refers to the 'passing over' of Jewish households during the last of the 10 plagues visited on the Egyptians before they were persuaded to free the Jews from slavery. During this time, observant Jews refrain from eating leavened bread, and partake of flat crackers, known as matzo.

Before the start of Passover, the house is thoroughly cleaned and all traces of leavened bread removed. This can be turned into a game for the children in which pieces of bread are deliberately hidden for them to find. In US Orthodox Jewish households, the days preceding Passover are an opportunity for 'spring cleaning'. The entire home must be made 'kosher for Passover'. As this is such a holy holiday, some families interpret the Jewish laws literally. This means that old household appliances, such as toasters or ovens, that might have been contaminated by leavened breads and less kosher food items may be either physically removed and new appliances purchased for the home or temporarily 'sold' to non-Jewish neighbors (they are not removed and no longer considered the property of the family, and are 'sold' back to the family after the holidays).

At the feast of Passover, the whole family eats a traditional meal called Seder, which has prescribed foods and a prescribed order. During the meal, those present drink four glasses of wine to recall the promises made to Moses by God. A fifth glass sits untouched on the table as a reminder of the belief that, at some point in the future, the prophet Elijah will return to earth at Passover to herald the start of the Messiah's reign on earth. The youngest child of the household then asks four standard questions and the head of the household tells everyone the story of the exodus in answering them. There are six dishes on a plate in the middle of the table. Two of them remain untouched (a roasted shankbone and an egg), but the others are tasted. Three matzah loaves recall the fact that when the Jews left Egypt, they did so with such speed that they could not wait for their loaves to rise and therefore took only unleavened bread. Maror or bitter herbs recall the bitterness of over 400 years of slavery in Egypt. Parsley dipped in vinegar or salt water is a reminder of the tears of the Hebrew slaves. A mixture of nuts, apple and wine – *haroset* – symbolizes the cement that the Jews were forced to use in building houses for the Egyptians.

Rites of passage

Circumcision is regarded as a religious obligation for parents of Jewish boys as a token of the covenant between the child and God. The tradition started when Abraham obeyed God's command to circumcise himself (at the age of 99 years) and all the male members of his household. Isaac, the first born son of a circumcised Jew, had his circumcision on the 8th day of life. Since then it has been traditional to circumcise boys on the 8th day of life irrespective of whether that day happens to be the Sabbath or even Yom Kippur. According to the Jewish calendar, a day begins at sunset on the preceding night, so if a boy was born on a Monday night his circumcision or *bris* would be on the following Tuesday. If the baby is in any way unwell or infirm, Jewish law dictates that the *bris* be postponed until he is well.

Brit milah is a religious ceremony performed by a *mohel* or ritual circumciser. It is usually performed in the home. Technically, the father is responsible for his son's circumcision, but the *mohel* acts as his representative. The only other person who must be present is the *sandek* or trusted assistant, usually the grandfather, who holds the baby during the procedure. The procedure is often undertaken without anesthetic, though a local anesthetic cream or wine may be used; how much pain a baby suffers by being circumcised with little or no anesthesia is controversial.

Some parents prefer to have their babies circumcised in a hospital setting because of concerns about anesthesia or cleanliness. (This does not have the same religious ceremony attached to it and is therefore regarded by some Jews as a poor substitute for a *bris* performed by a *mohel*.) In the UK and USA, most hospitals have at least one individual who will undertake circumcision on parental request. In the USA, some physicians have been trained as *mohels* to perform ritual circumcisions in the hospital setting. Circumcisions performed under Jewish law are to be made by a single cut; thus the Mogen clamp is used instead of the typical Gomco™ clamp or the Plastibell™ used for other circumcisions.

Bar mitzvah/bat mitzvah. At 12–13 years of age, a young person is regarded as being fully capable of participating in Jewish life. This transition is marked by the ceremonies of *bar mitzvah* for boys and *bat mitzvah* for girls. The boys spend months studying and memorizing verses from the Torah with the rabbi. A service in the synagogue is followed by a coming-of-age party for friends and family, which may be very lavish.

Family

The family and the family home are central to the Jewish faith. Celebrations throughout life will be shared not only with immediate family, but with the extended family and friends as well.

It is common for parents and the extended family to show great concern regarding marriage partners, particularly if anyone decides to 'marry out' (i.e. marry a non-Jew). In ultra-Orthodox communities in the USA, in which autosomal recessive genetic disease is a serious concern, some rabbis are taking on the role of matchmaker to supervise genetic testing and guide marriages between families with known carrier states.

Marriage within the Jewish community is a cause for much celebration. Weddings do not take place on festival days or on the Sabbath, which could violate the prohibition against work and travel, and the injunction against mixing one joy with another. For this reason, it is common for Jewish weddings to take place on Sundays.

Jewish wedding ceremonies take place under a bridal canopy or *chuppah* and comprise a number of rituals: the bride walks around the groom seven times to represent the 7 days of the creation of the world; the sharing of two cups of wine; the giving of the ring; the signing of the *Ketubah* (marriage contract) by two witnesses; the recitation of seven blessings; and the breaking of the glass symbolizing the destruction of the Temple in Jerusalem. The groom presents the bride with the *Ketubah*, which is often a beautiful piece of art that is prominently displayed in the new home. At Orthodox Jewish wedding receptions, men dance only with men and women are permitted to dance only with other women.

Divorce is an unhappy fact of life within Jewish circles as elsewhere. Traditionally, it was the prerogative of a man to initiate divorce proceedings and for a wife to agree or disagree, and then the matter would be decided by a religious court. There are strict rules that the rabbi follows in granting permission for a 'get' or divorce. In modern times, however, divorce is a civil proceeding and few couples seek any religious dispensation. In some liberal circles, there has been a move to recognize divorce in a sympathetic religious sense in order to help a couple achieve closure.

Dress

Unless a person is either Orthodox and wears a *yarmulke* (skullcap) or ultra-Orthodox, their Jewishness may go unnoticed. Ultra-Orthodox Jewish men and boys wear black trousers and waistcoat, covered with a black overcoat. Some wear breeches with knee-high white stockings. They shave their heads except for small areas at the front above their ears, which are left long and curly (as per directions in the book of Leviticus in the Torah). Men do not shave their beards, as proscribed by Jewish law. All wear *yarmulke* and men wear a brimmed black felt hat when they are outside. Prominent male members of the Orthodox community wear large, expensive mink hats.

Women from the ultra-Orthodox community are expected to dress modestly and never to show their hair to a man other than their husbands, as immodesty is regarded as a temptation to men to stray from their wives and thus represents a threat to family life. Women will usually wear long skirts and tops, which button up to the neck. They shave their heads and wear wigs or headscarves. Many women wear both wigs and hats when outside the home. However, if admitted to hospital, they will wear a head scarf or turban. Some will only wear hats on the Sabbath.

Although less strictly observant Jews may wear special items for prayer (see above), they are not worn in the street.

Food and drink

Food is a subject of great concern to many Jews. Dietary rules given to Moses by God and laid down in the bible are called *kashrut*. These laws are strict and represent a defining element for some Jews of what it means to be Jewish. For Orthodox Jews, they are non-negotiable, but for others, the rules are variably followed or disregarded; approximately 25–30% of US Jews claim to 'keep *kosher*'.

The laws of *kashrut* divide all edibles into *kosher* and *trafe*.

- *Kosher* means fit or proper and designates those things which are fit to eat.
- *Trafe* means torn or damaged and indicates those things that are not acceptable to eat.

Kosher is further subdivided into dairy (*milchig*), meat (*flayshig*) and neutral (*pareve*). *Kashrut* demands a complete separation of meat and dairy foods, but *pareve* foods such as fruit, nuts, seeds, vegetables, fish and eggs may be eaten with either meat or dairy foods. This has been interpreted over time to mean not only that meat and dairy should not be eaten together, but also that there should be complete separation of meat and dairy products in the kitchen. Thus, a *kosher* kitchen will have two sets of dishes and utensils, and even separate preparation areas, refrigerators and dishwasher racks.

Food products certified by rabbis or rabbinical organizations as *kosher* will be labeled with a mark called a *hekhsher* (or *hechsher*) – variable symbols according to the certifying rabbinical authority but which may include the letter 'K' or a letter 'U' within a small circle in the USA.

Fruit and vegetables. Everything that grows is both *kosher* and *pareve*. This means that all types of plants, fungi, vegetables, fruits, roots, nuts and seeds are permitted.

Fish that have scales, fins and gills are permitted. Non-*kosher* fish include shellfish, crustacea, eels, shark, whale and other sea mammals. Frog and octopus are also forbidden.

Meat. Animals that chew the cud and have cloven hooves are *kosher*; this includes cows, sheep, goat and deer. Animals that are forbidden include pigs, camels, donkeys and horses.

In order for meat to be *kosher*, it must not only be from a prescribed animal, but the animal must be slaughtered in a certain way by a certified butcher who is conversant with the religious laws regarding the production of meat and has the practical skills to carry them out. Following slaughter, the meat must be soaked in water, salted and soaked again to remove all traces of blood.

Fowl. Most domestic birds are regarded as *kosher* but, because they are meat, they must be slaughtered, inspected, soaked and prepared as above. Wild birds and birds of prey are forbidden, as are their eggs. Eggs from kosher birds are both *kosher* and *pareve*, although a single spot of blood within them renders them non-*kosher*.

Dairy products. All dairy products are permitted, but not at the same meal as beef. For example, ice cream will not be served at a wedding serving beef steak.

Alcohol. Kosher wine is that made under rabbinical supervision, though many Jews regard all wine as *kosher*. All beer, wine, grain and fruit alcohols are regarded as *kosher*, but some cream liqueurs are considered dairy products.

General health issues

Prescription medications are subject to *kosher* certification. There are even *kosher* prenatal vitamins for pregnant women. In general, any pill covered with a gelatin coating derived from *trafe* animal products is considered non-*kosher*. When deciding whether or not to take a medication, patients may be advised to consult their physician and rabbi to discuss the benefits and risks involved, and the possibility of alternative treatments.

Most hospitals provide *kosher* meals for patients on request. These are usually prepared outside the hospital by a Jewish caterer and packed ready for reheating when required.

The prevalence of the autosomal recessive gene responsible for Tay-Sachs disease (a progressive, neurological disorder resulting in death before 2 years of age in most cases) is particularly high in Ashkenazi Jews and their descendants. Awareness of the Tay-Sachs gene is generally high in Jewish populations and genetic testing is often done before considering possible marriage partners. Other autosomal recessive diseases that are found in the Jewish population have led several centers in the USA to offer 'Jewish Inheritible Disease' screening test panels.

Male patients may request not to have female healthcare providers to avoid physical contact with any woman that might be menstruating and considered 'unclean'. Similarly, husbands or fathers of female patients will not shake hands with female physicians or healthcare providers.

Contraception and reproduction

Children are regarded by Jews as a gift from God and to have them is both a blessing and commanded by the bible. Many Jews do not restrict themselves with regard to when they may have sexual intercourse or use contraception. Orthodox Jews, however, are far more rigorous and their interpretation of when sexual intercourse is permitted is in keeping with biblical orders to 'be fruitful and multiply'.

Orthodox Jews often do not use any formal contraception. Furthermore, women are regarded as 'unclean' until 7 days after the end of menstruation (on average, day 12–14 of the cycle). They then take a ritual bath and are allowed to resume sexual relations with their husbands. Menstrual irregularity or intermenstrual spotting, therefore, may lead to a number of difficulties; it may interfere with sexual relationships and also the ability to conceive.

Certain treatments are likely to be unacceptable to Orthodox Jewish women. These include any gynecologic medical procedure that is associated with vaginal bleeding, such as cervical biopsy, endometrial biopsy or 'Pap' (Papanicolau/cervical) smears, and anything with a contraceptive effect, even if it is not primarily being prescribed for that purpose. When dilemmas such as this arise, advice on the interpretation of Jewish law in unusual circumstances may be sought from religious leaders.

Since large families of five children or more are the norm in Orthodox Jewish communities, women will wish to deliver vaginally when possible. They will avoid primary and repeat cesarean deliveries, which may limit the number of children she can have and increase the likelihood of hysterectomy. They will also decline permanent tubal sterilization procedures even if it may be medically dangerous for the woman to get pregnant again.

Infertility. As in many other groups, infertility is becoming more common among Jewish couples. Factors contributing to this include marriage at a later age and women deferring childbearing until they have completed college studies and/or established their careers.

There is no objection to the use of fertility drugs from within the Jewish community. However, fertility treatment can lead to a high order multiple pregnancy and the difficult issue of selective reduction may arise. This is more problematic in the USA than in the UK, because of the different restrictions regarding the numbers of embryos which can be transferred after in-vitro fertilization. Although Judaism does not support abortion, apart from in exceptional circumstances, if selective reduction of a high multiple pregnancy gives the remaining fetuses a better chance of survival, it may be allowed under Jewish law.

Egg donation can present a dilemma for Jewish couples: some will wish the donor to be Jewish while others feel that it increases the possibility of committing incest either at the time or between offspring of the same donor in the future.

Abortion. Jewish tradition considers all life (including the life of a fetus) as sacred and does not permit abortion on request. However, Judaism does not regard the fetus as a full human being so abortion is permitted under some circumstances, particularly for medical reasons. In general, when abortion is necessary, it must take place before the first 40 days, when the fetus is referred to as 'mere water'; however, more progressive Jews believe that the fetus does not acquire a soul until after delivery. Maternal health and safety are considered a priority over that of the unborn fetus.

Strong views about abortion prevent many women from even considering the idea of prenatal testing for conditions such as Down's syndrome and some will even wish not to have an anomaly scan. In general, these strong views apply to women from the Orthodox community, but as ever, there is a spectrum of opinion on these matters. Some women will wish to be tested so that they can make adequate preparation for the birth of an affected child. Gentle inquiry regarding prenatal testing and the views of a woman and her partner is better than preconceived ideas that may result in either denial of aspects of medical care or unintended insult.

Birth. Orthodox Jewish men generally do not come to the labor and delivery rooms with their wives, because the blood from the genital tract associated with the delivery process is considered 'unclean'. An Orthodox Jewish woman who is about to give birth will typically have another female relative or friend with them in the delivery room, while the husband stands outside the room in rhythmic prayer.

Sexuality

As with other faiths, the union of a man and a woman in marriage and the production of children are highly prized . Although traditional Jewish thinking does not permit homosexuality on the basis that it does not allow procreation, there is a recognized movement within liberal Jewish circles that represents lesbian and gay Jews.

Death

Jewish law and custom regarding death and mourning are based on the principle of respect both for the dead person and also for their bereaved relatives. Mourners are given a structure to help them with the funeral arrangements and for the period thereafter, which encourages the expression rather than repression of grief.

Jewish law does not permit autopsy on the grounds that it is a desecration of the body and disrespectful. Clearly, if an autopsy is required by law, it is a different matter. In this case, performing an autopsy and releasing the body to the family as quickly as possible is imperative. Saving a life takes precedence over all other Jewish laws and autopsy, organ donation and organ preservation may all be permitted under this clause, usually after discussion with a rabbi.

The body of the dead person is treated with respect. The eyes and mouth are closed, a candle is lit as a symbol of the soul and a window opened to allow the soul to escape. The body is washed and clothed in a simple white shroud. According to Jewish custom, the body must not be left alone and this role may be fulfilled by a family member or friend, or someone from a Jewish funeral parlor may be asked to deputize. The body should be buried as quickly as possible, although funerals are not permitted on the Sabbath or festival days. A funeral may also be delayed to allow family members to be present.

The Torah describes the 'renting (tearing) of clothes' at funerals. This practice is continued today by some who will tear their jacket lapels if male, or a blouse or dress if female. Alternatively, some people wear a torn black ribbon on their lapel as a sign of mourning.

Jewish law specifically prohibits cremation. Cremation is believed to interfere with the natural process of decomposition and the 'return to the earth' of a dead body, which should take place. In modern times, cremation also has sinister overtones as it reminds many Jews of the Holocaust.

The 7 days following burial are known as *shiva*. During *shiva*, mourners receive visitors who come to express condolence into the house. Since the purpose of mourning is to allow expression of grief and sorrow, it is not customary to send flowers to a Jewish house of mourning as they are seen as something to beautify and cheer up a place. However, food baskets are welcomed.

The 30 days after the burial, which include *shiva*, are called *sheloshim*. During this phase, mourners return to work and start to return to normality. After the 30th day, all outward signs of mourning are dispensed with except for those who have lost a parent who may continue to mourn officially for a full Jewish year following the burial.

Jewish cemeteries are usually separate from grave sites of non-Jewish dead. Those that have passed away are remembered by the placement of stones on the gravestone, and the naming of newborn children with similar names.

In contemporary life and especially in more liberal circles, many of the old traditions of mourning have been entirely dispensed with or have been watered down considerably. It is interesting, however, that it has become increasingly well recognized that mourning appropriately at the time of the death can help to prevent repressed grief, which can seriously impair emotional and/or physical health in later life.

Key points – Judaism

- The Jewish faith is around 4000 years old with large numbers of contemporary followers concentrated in Israel, but with significant numbers in New York city and the UK, as well as other countries around the world.
- Jewish law is defined by the Torah – part of the holy book of the faith, and contains directions regarding food, hairstyles, headcoverings, clothing and worship.
- Prescription medicines are subject to *kosher* certification. Most hospitals will provide *kosher* meals for patients on request.
- Men may request a male physician to avoid physical contact with any woman who might be menstruating and would therefore be considered 'unclean'.
- Jewish law does not permit autopsy, as desecration of the body is seen as disrespectful. If required by law, release of the body as quickly as possible is imperative.
- Circumcision for baby boys on the 8th day of life is required by Jewish law.

Adherents to the Sikh faith number around 24 million worldwide, representing around 0.39% of the world's population. There are approximately half a million Sikhs in North America and a quarter of a million in Europe. Sikhism is derived from Hinduism and has many common attributes. Geographically, Sikhism has its origins in the 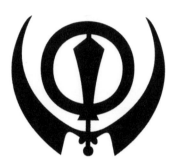 Punjab region of Northern India. Part of the Punjab became annexed to Pakistan during the partition of 1947 and a large number of Sikhs moved away from the area. The partition remains a source of conflict to this day. While the majority of Sikhs still live in the Punjab, there are large Sikh communities in the UK and USA.

Belief in one God and the teachings of the 10 Gurus is at the heart of Sikhism. The first guru was Guru Nanak, who was born into a wealthy Hindu family in 1469 in the city of Talwindi (now Nankana Sahib in modern Pakistan). Guru Nanak was an unusually intelligent child and had reservations about aspects of both the Hindu and Muslim faiths. At 30 years of age, he was bathing in the river and felt himself drawn up to God, where he was given a cup of sweet nectar to drink. Although his friends and family believed he had drowned, he returned to them 3 days later and told them that God had called him to be a Guru. From then on he traveled widely and preached his message. He believed that God was neither a Hindu nor a Muslim and his message adopted aspects of both religions while rejecting others. Accordingly, the Sikh faith is based on the following principles.

- There is one God who is with them in the world but is also overseer of all the world.
- There is a continual cycle of birth, death and rebirth through which everyone must pass in their quest for the ultimate aim.

- The ultimate aim of each person's soul is to be reabsorbed into the God from whence they came.
- Those who live by God must exercise self-discipline and live according to a certain moral code. Most importantly, they must be humble and always at the service of others.

Guru Nanak was followed by nine other Gurus, who developed the Sikh faith over the next 2 centuries.

Although the founders of Sikhism date back to the 1400s, the religion was not defined until the early part of the last century. In 1925, the Sikh Gurudwaras Act in India defined Sikhs as those who believed in the 10 Gurus and the Guru Granth Sahib (or Adi Granth – the holy book), and were not lapsed members. A meeting in Amritsar in 1931 further defined Sikh belief and practice. From then on Sikhs would be those who believed in one God and the teachings of the 10 Gurus and the Adi Granth, Sikhs would accept the importance and meaning of the holy nectar, Sikhs would live in Sikh communities accepting the values of and practicing according to the traditions of that community, and Sikhs would not belong to any other religion.

The aim of a Sikh is to live a good life so that the chances of the soul being reunited with God are increased. Sikhs do not believe in impurity at birth or death, but that actions in previous lives may affect the present and that the only way out of this cycle is to listen to the word of God, perform good deeds and keep good company. A further belief is that all humans suffer as a result of failure to appreciate God's creation and failure to control the mind.

Sikhs are not encouraged to become ascetics and cut themselves off from the world. A Sikh's way of life is described as neither asceticism nor hedonism, but somewhere between the two along the 'middle path'. While a life of contemplation is compatible with the Sikh faith, the abandonment of work and family responsibilities is discouraged.

A strong work ethic pervades the Sikh faith and idleness is unacceptable. The acquisition of wealth through hard work is acceptable, though overt displays of affluence and hoarding of assets are not. Sikhs are obliged to share any excess wealth with those who are needy.

All people are seen as equal in the eyes of God according to the Sikh faith. For this reason, men and women have equal status within the religion and anyone is welcome in a Gurudwara (the Sikh place of worship) and to partake of the free meal offered there.

Astrology, superstition and the worship of tombs and temples are not acceptable in Sikhism.

Worship

The Gurudwara, or temple, is usually a simple building with plain walls and a raised area at the front where the Guru Granth Sahib is placed during worship. Shoes must be removed before entering the Gurudwara. Men's heads are covered by their turbans and women cover their heads with a scarf. There are no seats and worshippers sit cross-legged on the floor, ensuring that their feet are not pointing towards the scriptures. Men and women sit in separate places in the main body of the Gurudwara, but men and women are equally able to lead prayers.

The main day of worship is Sunday, though other services take place throughout the week. Private prayers may be offered at any time, but collective worship is an obligation for Sikhs. Traditionally, Sikhs rise early, bathe and then undertake a morning meditation using a set prayer. There are also set prayers for other times in the day. The Westernization of many societies with its introduction of shift patterns can make adherence to prayers and meditation difficult.

Scripture

Sikhs treat their holy book, the Guru Granth Sahib, as a living Guru. It is written in Gurmukhi, a form of Hindi used in the Middle Ages, and contains the actual words spoken by the 10 Gurus written as hymns of varying lengths. A trained reader of the Guru Granth Sahib uses a special fan called a *chauri* made of nylon or yak hair embedded in bone or silver or occasionally peacock feathers. This is waved over the Guru Granth Sahib as a mark of respect and represents the respectful fanning of a Guru in a hot country.

A Guru Granth Sahib is kept in many Sikh homes, preferably in a room of its own and upstairs if the family live in a house. This is to facilitate quiet study and contemplation, as well as to avoid people walking over the place where it is stored, which is regarded as disrespectful. The holy text will be opened during the morning and put to rest (closed and laid respectfully) after sunset each day, remembering that this book is treated as if it were the embodiment of a person. When a Guru Granth Sahib is too old to be used any longer, it is cremated and the ashes are scattered in a local river in much the same way as one might cremate and scatter the ashes of a person.

Rites of passage

Khalsa is the name given by Guru Gobind Singh to all Sikhs who have been baptized or initiated into the Sikh faith. Initiation into the *Khalsa* takes place in the Gurudwara. At the ceremony, the initiates pledge to be true to the way of the *Khalsa* (symbolized by the Khanda, see figure on page 76) and drink nectar (*amrit*), which is prepared by stirring sugar crystals into water using a double-edged sword in an iron bowl. This initiation can take place at any age, except in the very young, and is not regarded as a sacrament. In addition to the ceremony, *Khalsa* must wear the five 'Ks':

- *kesh* – uncut hair and beards as a sign of devotion to God
- *kirpan* – the sword symbolic of the willingness to fight against spiritual and physical oppression
- *kangha* – a comb necessary for cleanliness and good personal hygiene, which is very important to Sikhs
- *kara* – a steel bracelet, which signifies that God is one and that the link between God and believer is unbreakable
- *kachera* – traditional shorts worn to show that the person is always ready to defend the Sikh faith.

For a person who has broken any of the vows (e.g. cut their hair, eaten *halal* meat, committed adultery), the initiation ceremony may be performed again, but only if it is believed that the person is truly sorry for what they have done and is renewing their vows wholeheartedly.

Festivals

The three main festivals are: Diwali, Holi and Baisakhi. Diwali, the Festival of Lights, derives from Hindu culture (see page 31). The festival of Holi, which celebrates the triumph of good over bad, is very popular in Northern India and is associated with much merrymaking and general excess. It precedes the Sikh festival of Hola Mohalla (meaning attack and place of attack), which was established by Guru Gobind Singh as a celebration of music, readings, religion, poetry reading, martial displays and mock battles.

Baisakhi is the only festival to occur on a fixed date each year (13th April) as it is based on the solar year. It marks the beginning of the year in Northern India. It is of particular importance to Sikhs as on this day in 1699 Guru Gobind Singh brought the Sikh faith into being as a separate entity. For this reason, Sikhs are often initiated into the faith at Baisakhi, though there is no objection to this taking place at other times of the year. Other celebrations in the Sikh calendar are the Gurpurbs, which mark holy days in honor of the various Gurus.

Family

Sikhs may have a large extended family, which includes all members of the Sikh community. The elders are valued and cared for by their family. Arranged marriages are still common, though parents are likely to allow their children greater freedom of choice of partner than previously. It is likely that the prospective couple will meet to decide whether they wish to pursue a long-term relationship. It is preferable to select a marriage partner from the same caste or social group; 'marrying out', where a Sikh chooses a partner from a different religious or cultural background or someone from a lower social group, is discouraged. Protection of honor is important and sex outside a committed relationship is discouraged even in the more liberal West.

Traditional marriage ceremonies last 5 days and take place in the home town or village of the bride's family, who are responsible for the entire celebration with its attendant expense. The bride then goes to live with her husband's family. This extended family arrangement within the same household is still common even in Westernized families, though increasing numbers of young couples are choosing to live a more nuclear existence.

Divorce is as much a sad fact of life for Sikhs as for any other group. While divorce is not ideal, marriage to an unsuitable partner is regarded as worse and may result in the individuals being castigated by family

and friends.

Dress

The most obvious form of traditional Sikh attire is the turban worn by
men. This is a head-covering formed from the elaborate winding of a
single piece of cloth and may be of any color. Both men and women do
not cut their hair. When boys are considered old enough to wear a
turban, typically at around the age of 12 years, a celebration is often
held in the Gurudwara. Until that time, boys' hair is tied in a top-knot
and may be covered with a small piece of fabric. If a turban has to be
removed for medical reasons, most Sikh men will want their head and
hair covered with a cloth. The turban should be handled with care and
held using two hands. If possible, it should be left near the patient and
should not be placed in a bag with other clothing or allowed to touch
the floor.

Although men and women are equal, women are expected to cover
their legs. Traditional dress for both men and women involves wearing
special shorts as an undergarment beneath their clothes, which are
usually loose, often in the form of pajama-type trousers called *salvars*,
with a long shirt over the top that reaches to the knees. If the *kachera*
(shorts) have to be removed for medical examinations or childbirth,
discuss keeping them around one leg instead of removing them.

Women will generally cover their heads with a *dupatta* for modesty,
except in the home. In the UK and elsewhere in the Western world,
many Sikhs are giving up traditional forms of dress in preference to
Western-style clothes.

Food and drink

Sikhs have very few restrictions regarding food. Some Sikhs eat meat
more regularly than others, but some actively choose not to eat meat
and discourage others from doing so. The food prepared in the
communal kitchen at the Gurudwara is always vegetarian so as not to
offend anyone. The traditional Sikh diet is a reflection of the foods
found in abundance in the Sikh homeland in the Punjab region of India
and consists of cereals, grains, fresh vegetables and fruit. Very little meat
is consumed in the Punjab except during celebrations, such as weddings.

Sikhs who eat meat may choose not to eat *halal* meat (i.e. killed
according to Muslim law). This practice has its roots in the days of

the Moghul rule in India when Sikhism was developing and *halal* meat was used to effect conversions to Islam. As a consequence, Sikhs were commanded by Guru Gobind Singh not to eat *halal* meat as a protest against the differential treatment of those who were Muslims and those who were not. Elders of the community may, as part of their increasing devotion to the faith, rescind eating meat in the pursuit of bodily purity.

Alcohol is forbidden by the Sikh faith though this is an injunction that is widely ignored.

General health issues

The body of a Sikh is regarded as a temple of the soul and as such must be kept in good condition. This means abstaining from intoxicants, but also feeding the body well and allowing it adequate rest. Thus, leisure is a requirement of the Sikh faith so long as it does not harm others. Gambling, drinking, and immoral entertainment are not permitted, nor is the keeping of undesirable company. Smoking is also forbidden.

When taking care of Sikh patients in the hospital setting, same-sex caregivers, including physicians, are preferred, particularly for women. It is important to protect the modesty of female patients and leave the body covered as much as possible. Family members are likely to want to stay with a relative who is hospitalized and should be allowed to participate in their care as much as possible to make the patient feel at ease.

The five Ks are worn at all times, even during hospitalization, when ill at home and when washing. Healthcare providers should consult the patient or other family members before removing any of these items for hospitalization or before surgical procedures. Cutting/shaving of hair while the Sikh is hospitalized should be avoided; if it is medically necessary in preparation for surgery, the patient or family should be consulted.

Sikhs prefer to take baths rather than showers; baths are usually taken daily at dawn, and followed by meditation and prayer.

Sikhs generally have no issues with accepting blood transfusions or receiving organ transplants if medically indicated.

Contraception and reproduction

Women may consider themselves unclean during menstruation. There are, however, no specific rules regarding reproduction or contraception and all methods are open to Sikhs.

Infertility. In the past, a woman who was unable to bear children would have been likely to have been left by her husband, but this has changed with the advent of reproductive technology. Nevertheless, not producing a son and heir to the family name is regarded as a source of sadness and even shame on a woman. Artificial insemination is permissible in Sikh religion as long as the sperm is from the husband.

Abortion. Most Sikhs believe that life begins at conception, so if conception has taken place it would be a sin to destroy life by elective abortion. However, the Sikh code of conduct does not directly prohibit abortion or attempt to address any other bioethical issues. Abortion is treated in much the same way as in most faiths; it is discouraged but accepted as the lesser of two evils if continuing with the pregnancy would be to the significant detriment of the woman, the unborn child or her family. However, the cultural preference for male offspring is leading to a growing desire to abort female fetuses.

Birth. Children are considered a gift from God in Sikh culture. Traditionally, the father will whisper the *Mul Mantra* (Guru Nanak's first poetic statement) into the newborn's ear as soon as possible following birth. The mother may need to be secluded for a period of 13–40 days following delivery, while she is still experiencing vaginal bleeding. This is considered a time of impurity.

There are no special community ceremonies at the time of the birth but family and friends will gather on an appointed day at the Gurudwara sometime after the birth for the naming ceremony. At this ceremony, the Guru Granth Sahib will be opened at random and the first letter of the first word of the hymn that appears forms the initial letter of the child's name. Once the name has been chosen, it is announced to the congregation. The ceremony is one of thanksgiving for the birth of the child.

While the birth of a daughter is not regarded as a tragedy, it is not greeted with the same elation and exchange of congratulations and presents between relatives and friends as that of a son. Girls are still seen as something of an expensive liability.

Sexuality

As with other faiths, there is emphasis on the union of a man and a woman in marriage and the bearing of children. Homosexuality is not encouraged nor necessarily condoned.

Death

When death is approaching, the dying person is encouraged to say *'wahe guru, wahe guru'* (wonderful Lord) several times. Relatives or close friends in attendance may recite a hymn of peace or other text. Scriptures will be read and hymns sung during the last hours of a Sikh's life.

When the person has died, mourners are discouraged from wailing and weeping by being reminded that it is God's will that we are born and must die. Hope, rather than sadness, usually characterizes the death of a Sikh. Expressions of grief for one who has lived a happy and long life are limited or not seen at all. It is believed that outward expressions of grief (e.g. crying) will interfere with the peaceful departure of the dying person. Expressions of grief may be more liberal if a person dies early in life or from some unnatural cause.

Families will usually accept requests for autopsy, but it is generally not desirable unless required by law. Surviving Sikh family members may consider organ transplantation or donation acceptable.

The body of a Sikh is preferably cremated as soon after death as possible, generally within 24 hours. Stillborn and young babies may be buried. The body is first washed and dressed in the symbols of faith. The washing of the body is undertaken by members of the family of the same sex as the deceased. Limbs are straightened. The face is cleaned and the eyes and mouth closed. The head is wrapped in a turban. If no family member is available, the head of the deceased should be kept covered. All hair should be left untrimmed. The body is then dressed in new clothes, a white shroud or solid white sheet. Items which were meaningful to the deceased may be placed inside the coffin. The body may be taken to the family home for family members to pay their respects or may be viewed at the hospital mortuary or at the funeral parlor.

During the cremation, prayers are recited, a few pages of the scriptures are read and ceremonial food is distributed. The mourners then take their leave of the family but may continue to visit them in their home for several days afterwards. The ashes are collected from the crematorium the day after the cremation and are usually scattered on a river or stream. Sikhs regard the river Ganges as holy and scattering of ashes into this river is particularly special; however, if this is not practical, a nearby river or stream may be substituted. Sikhs are not permitted to erect any monuments to the dead, but are encouraged to view their dead loved ones as being with them through their deeds. After about 10 days, the reading of the appropriate scripture is completed and there is a final gathering after which there is no further formal mourning.

Key points – Sikhism

- The Sikh faith was founded in the 16th century by Guru Nanak in what is now the Punjab region of India.
- The faith encourages doing good rather than carrying out rituals and stresses the importance of the internal spiritual state of the individual.
- Physical evidence of belonging to the Sikh faith is denoted by the five 'Ks': uncut hair (*kesh*); a steel bracelet (*kara*); a wooden comb (*kanga*); cotton underwear (*kachera*); and a steel sword (*kirpan*).
- If the turban, worn by Sikh men, has to be removed for medical reasons, it should be handled with care and with two hands. It should not be placed in a bag or on the floor, and should be left as near to the patient as possible.
- A same-sex physician is usually preferred, especially by Sikh women.
- There is a cultural preference for male offspring.

Traditional Chinese Religion and its associated Oriental health beliefs and practices is not an organized, unified system of religion in the traditional sense. There are no religious leaders, headquarters, founders or denominations. Sometimes labeled as Chinese Universalism, the cultural beliefs/rituals and health practices of many people of Chinese ancestry are more appropriately known as Traditional Chinese Religion. Their attitude and approach towards the maintenance of health and the treatment of disease is commonly known as Traditional Chinese Medicine (TCM). These practices and beliefs are generally based on a balance of hot and cold, yin and yang principles, and/or harmony with the universe, hence the term 'Chinese Universalists'.

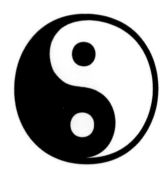

Traditional Chinese Religion was heavily influenced by the Buddhist and Hindu religions in pre-Communist China. Although other religions have affected traditional Chinese beliefs and practices, Chinese 'religion' is a complex amalgamation of four historic traditions or philosophies:

- Confucianism
- Taoism
- Chinese folk religion
- Buddhism.

The religious outlook of most Chinese people (despite the ban on religious practices in China following the Communist Revolution in 1949) consists of a combination of beliefs and practices taken from these four traditions. It is rare for only one set of beliefs and practices to be followed to the exclusion of the others and this has, in turn, been adopted by other peoples in Asia, South Asia, and South East Asia.

Philosophy

Confucianism sets rules of behavior to promote social harmony by dictating social duties and proper interpersonal behaviors and defining social hierarchies. The family is at the center of all social responsibilities and comes before the individual. The father is the undisputed head of the family and treated with filial piety. The eldest son has the obligation to take care of elderly parents and the family, which includes making healthcare decisions.

Control of one's emotions, demonstration of restraint, obedience to authority, personal sacrifice for the benefit of the family and saving 'face' are highly valued and important principles even during illness in the hospital setting. For example, because traditional Chinese values place the family and society before the individual, attempted suicide does not necessarily carry the psychiatric stigma of mental illness as it does in Western society, especially if it was associated with duty or family loyalty.

The tradition of deference to authority may also lead to misunderstanding; for example, when patients nod their heads, they may be simply deferring to authority (the physician) and not indicating understanding and agreement. It is therefore important to be sure that the patient understands what is being said and is not just being polite. However, when communication is clear, patients with traditional Chinese beliefs are quite compliant with medical treatment.

Taoism is an ancient Chinese religion that is not entirely distinct from Confucianism or Chinese folk religion. Taoism is characterized by an awareness of man's close relationship with nature and the universe, a cyclical view of time (not linear as in Western culture), veneration or worship of ancestors and the ideas of heaven and spiritual harmony. Taoist beliefs include the concept that life is a balance of opposites in the universe – the yin and yang, good and evil, light and darkness – all of which are the double manifestations of the single, eternal cosmic principal: the Tao (Dao).

Also important in Taoism is the concept of heaven (T'ien), which is sometimes described in terms of an impersonal power or fate or letting nature take its course, and also known as the Tao or 'the way'. Taoists strongly believe in promoting health and vitality through the Five Elements, and the development of virtue by seeking compassion, moderation and humility.

The Taoist model of disease involves disharmony in the body's forces, a fatalistic view of health and herbal medicines which can be used to restore that balance. Followers of Traditional Chinese Religion tend to favor a crisis-oriented system of care in which, except for vaccinations, preventive medicine is virtually ignored (i.e. illness is a result of fate).

Yin and Yang. The Yin and Yang (see figure, page 86) is the general law of opposing forces.

- Yin is defined as 'female', a negative force and cold energy.
- Yang is defined as 'male', a positive force and hot energy.

The well-being of man, woman and child requires that these Yin and Yang forces be in balance. Illness results from an imbalance of the forces. Foods can be classified as 'hot' or 'cold' (this does not refer to the actual temperature) and a proper balance is required to maintain health. Illnesses and treatments are also considered as 'hot' or 'cold' and an illness will require a treatment of the opposite category to restore balance.

For example, pregnancy is normally considered a 'hot' state and 'yang' forces are consumed during the birthing process. Therefore, in the postpartum period, the 'cold' forces are out of balance and the woman requires replenishment of her 'yang' energy. During the traditional 30 days of postpartum confinement, the new mother should not be exposed to air conditioning ('cold'), no matter how warm she may feel, and should be fed foods such as chicken in sesame oil ('hot') to replace her Yang. Contrary to the Western concepts of a well-balanced diet, foods that contain green leafy vegetables are considered 'cold' in TCM, and are avoided during pregnancy and the postpartum period.

The color of Western medications can also be interpreted as 'hot' or 'cold'. Some patients with 'hot' diseases of Yang will refuse to take red ('hot')-colored pills or capsules.

Five Element Theory consists of the relationship between wood, fire, earth, metal and water. The five elements represent the major organs of the body:

- water = kidneys
- wood = liver
- fire = heart
- earth = spleen and pancreas
- metal = lungs.

The elements and organs are also linked to personality traits and disease states in an attempt to understand how the mind and body affect health. The essential premise of the Five Element Theory is that these basic elements of nature generate and regulate the 'chi' (vital energy) that controls health. Based on the Five Element Theory, each elemental force generates or creates the next element in a creative sequence:

- water generates wood by growing trees
- wood begets fire by burning
- fire generates earth by creating ashes
- earth generates metal by mining
- metal generates water by condensation.

These relationships are then applied to the human body in which each organ is responsible for providing the energy to the next organ in the cycle:

- the kidneys (water) support the liver (wood)
- the liver (wood) supports the heart (fire)
- the heart (fire) supports the spleen and pancreas (earth)
- the spleen and pancreas (earth) supports the lungs (metal)
- the lungs (metal) support the kidneys (water).

Conversely, the basic elements and organs can regulate or oppose other elemental forces; for example, water puts out fire, wood controls earth, fire melts metal, earth controls water and a metal axe can cut wood.

This theory is used to explain how the internal organs of the body are regulated by following the analogies of the elements; for example, the lungs control the liver, the heart controls the lungs, the kidneys control the heart, the spleen and pancreas control the kidneys, and the liver controls the spleen and pancreas. Thus, someone who feels tearful and sad, has 'metal' characteristics, which may indicate a lung imbalance. Using the Five Element Theory, the patient would be advised to avoid spicy foods, perform exercises that strengthen the lungs and have acupuncture treatments to promote 'chi' to the lungs.

Buddhism. Some Buddhist religious principles have been incorporated into TCM, even though the patients may not be practicing Buddhists. Like Confucianism, Buddhist teachings emphasize 'face' or dignity, and an individual's wrongdoing causes immediate family to lose face. Patients may therefore not admit or realize they have health problems, especially mental health problems, as they may bring shame on their families.

Other important teachings and beliefs include the concept of 'karma' and the idea that the development of disease is determined by destiny and not preventable.

Chinese folk religion is a combination of superstition, feng shui ('wind-water' or geomancy), numerology and word play. Many of these traditions have primarily been passed down by word of mouth. The color red is considered lucky, and the color white represents death. Chinese characters are considered symbols for the words they represent. Positive characters may be hung upside down to bring good luck and not tempt karma.

Feng shui is the practice of aligning buildings, furniture and other man-made structures to formations in nature such as mountains, lakes, oceans and trees – hence the term 'wind-water'. Feng shui masters, who have studied the harmonious placement of man-made objects, have also evolved to serve as a type of fortune-teller and advisor for those seeking additional folk religious wisdom.

Word play with homonyms that represent auspicious words is common, especially with numbers. For example, 8 August 2008 (8-8-08) is an auspicious date for weddings and births, so banquet halls and maternity wards, are expected be full worldwide.

Traditional Chinese Medicine

The practice of TCM can be organized into two broad categories:
- self/patient administered
- practitioner administered.

Self-administered health practices include meditation, exercise that cultivates the 'chi' (as in tai chi), general exercise, diet and nutrition. Practitioner-administered health practices include cupping and other manual manipulative techniques, moxibustion (burning herbs on the body), acupuncture and herbal medicine.

Cupping is the old traditional practice of applying cups made of plastic, ceramic, glass, horn or bamboo under suction to the patient's back for the purpose of encouraging chi and blood circulation in the body, and to detoxify the organs by drawing out impurities through the pores. There are two types of cupping procedure: stationary or moving. Stationary cupping involves applying several cups over sites of injury or acupuncture points and leaving them on suction for a period of time. Moving cupping procedures involve sliding the cups up and down the back, and around the scapula with massage oil to stimulate the flow of chi. Cups can also be placed over an inserted acupuncture needle for deeper stimulation.

Moxibustion involves the application of heat to relieve pain and create an overall sense of well-being by burning herbs, such as dried mugwort, rolled into a cigar-shaped stick over the affected parts of the body. Some forms of moxibustion involve placing the burning herbs directly onto the skin (scarring). Non-scarring forms of moxibustion include placing the burning herbs on top of an acupuncture needle for the heat to be transmitted deeper into the body or holding the burning moxibustion stick close to the skin without burning it.

The burning of the moxa is believed to warm the acupuncture points and expel the cold forces from the body. The burning of the moxa releases a pungent odor and a great deal of smoke, which may be irritating to patients with reactive airway disease.

Acupuncture is an ancient form of healing developed in China that involves the placement of solid, hair-thin needles that are inserted no more than 1 cm deep to activate 2000 or more acupuncture points distributed around the body. These acupuncture points are connected by 20 pathways, called meridians, which conduct the 'chi'.

Acupuncture is believed to keep the balance between yin and yang, thus allowing the normal flow of 'chi' and restoring health to the mind and body.

The needles are so fine that they do not draw blood; however, persons with a tendency to bruise or known hemophiliacs should consider alternatives to acupuncture.

The World Health Organization has recognized the ability of acupuncture to treat a variety of ailments: neuromuscular disorders, psychological disorders (e.g. depression, anxiety), gastrointestinal disorders (e.g. ulcers, diarrhea) and respiratory disorders (e.g. sinusitis, emphysema).

Worship

Traditional Chinese Religion does not require any formal forms of worship, since it is not an organized religion. Some practitioners may, however, visit Taoist or Buddhist temples to pray and burn incense.

Many people of Chinese ancestry have small altars in their own homes for the purpose of ancestor worship. The altars normally include a photograph of the deceased and a small shrine. The practice of ancestor worship most commonly consists of making food offerings of fruits and vegetables to the deceased to provide for them in the afterlife. Money (or pieces of paper representing money) is sometimes burned to provide money for dead ancestors. Family members bow and hold their hands together in prayer before the altar and photos to pay respect to the deceased.

Although there are several well-known Chinese Gods in Chinese mythology and folk religion, they are not worshipped, but represent a cultural identity.

Scripture

There are no written texts dictating how believers should behave. The rituals and traditions are passed down by family tradition and practice from generation to generation. The only rites of passage that are celebrated or acknowledged are birth, marriage and death. There are no 'coming of age' celebrations as in other cultures.

Family

Prior to the Communist Revolution in mainland China, large families were the mainstay of Asian culture. Male offspring are highly prized to carry on the family name so the more sons a family has, the more honor the family has.

As dictated by Confucian doctrine, responsibility to parents and family takes precedence over self-interest. The individual is expected to sacrifice him or herself for the good of the parents or the family honor. This respect for elders or filial piety may lead to a younger, but responsible, adult member of the family to unilaterally decide to not inform family members of illness to 'protect' them.

The decision maker for the family is traditionally the older son or husband. This responsible family member may be reluctant to place elderly parents or grandparents in long-term care and may avoid discussion about advance directives in making decisions for medical care.

Male children often receive preferential treatment or hold a place of honor in the family, especially first-born males, because they are expected to support the family and carry on the family name. Female offspring are not as valued because they marry into the husband's family and become their responsibility. However, with acculturation, daughters as well as sons are encouraged to excel. A good education and academic success are highly valued. Parents may be self-sacrificing to provide a better life for their children, including having several jobs or operating a small family business to save money for their children to have a college education.

Chinese weddings are extremely elaborate affairs. As well as wishing the bride and groom good luck and fertility, the toasts given at these weddings demonstrate the academic and financial successes of the two families. During the wedding banquet, the bride has an opportunity to show off her evening gowns with at least three changes of clothes. Modern brides may wear the Western white wedding gown; however, the traditional Chinese bride dresses in red, the color of good luck. The bride is not allowed to have white flowers (the color of death) in her wedding bouquet or the banquet decorations.

Divorce is generally frowned upon in Asian society. In ancient China, men were allowed to take more than one wife or have concubines to increase the size of the family and the number of sons.

Food and drink

There are no prohibitions on food and drink. Alcohol is permissible, although many Chinese Asians suffer from alcohol dehydrogenase deficiency and may find alcohol consumption unpleasant. Many Chinese Asians are also lactose intolerant. The Chinese Asian diet is typically high in salt, low in fat and low in roughage. Meats and seafood are considered bountiful, while vegetables are less valued. Some Asians will not eat pork or beef due to Buddhist and Hindu influences. For most Chinese Asians, however, there are no limitations to any animals, organs, fruits or vegetables in their diet, no matter how exotic. Most Chinese avoid eating uncooked vegetables and salads.

For those believing in the 'hot' and 'cold' theory or the Five Element Theory, different types of foods and drinks may be avoided or preferred to maintain the balance of 'chi'. The Chinese have a tendency to feed their children generously, especially male offspring. Overweight children are perceived as being healthier and represent the bounty of the family.

Family members prefer to bring appropriate foods from home for patients in hospital. Diabetic diets may not be compatible with 'hot' and 'cold' diets, and special counseling with dieticians may be required.

Dress

Most Chinese Asians dress very conservatively. Men keep their upper bodies covered regardless of heat or humidity. Most men are clean-shaven. Women should be appropriately covered to protect their modesty and short pants are frowned upon; however, younger generations have become more Westernized.

Festivals

There are no official religious festivals for the Chinese. Many of the festivals they celebrate come from folk traditions. The most important holiday is Chinese New Year which is based on the lunar calendar. Family members return home for many days of feasting. The banquets traditionally consist of a fowl (chicken or duck) or fish with its head and tail on the platter, representing the beginning of the new year and end of the old year, foods with nuts or pips representing the seed for the new year, and long noodles symbolizing a long life for all.

Other festivals include the Lantern Festival (which follows Chinese New Year), the Dragon Boat Festival and the Moon Festival (which celebrates the harvest). Families will individually celebrate the anniversary of the deaths of parents and grandparents by making offerings at home shrines. This is not a time for weeping or grieving, but celebration and honoring the importance of the ancestors.

General health issues

Chinese patients generally avoid going to see doctors, especially for preventive medicine. They will consult doctors only if there is a health concern and generally avoid interventions. The doctor-patient relationship is often very formal, which may conflict with the Western concept of the physician working with the patient as a partner rather than an authority figure. Patients prefer to be addressed as Mr or Mrs rather than by their first name. Patients will feel uncomfortable about physical contact with either family members or healthcare providers. Public displays of affection such as hand-holding, kissing or hugging are frowned upon, depending on the degree of acculturation. Physicians, as authority figures, are expected to make a rapid diagnosis and give instructions. Diagnostic tests are considered bothersome.

Many less acculturated Chinese immigrants may believe that Western medications are too strong and may not take prescribed doses. Chinese immigrants are also very frugal, and will cut medications in half to make the prescriptions last longer. They often look for bargains, less expensive substitutes or 'getting something for free'. Although taking Government assistance is generally frowned upon by the Chinese in the USA, food stamps and free coupons for pregnant women and children are considered a bonus.

In traditional Chinese culture, somatization is considered an acceptable way to express emotional distress and obtain attention, rather than an indication of mental illness. The patient may sometimes be perceived as a hypochondriac, but it is a form of communication. Dramatic comments such as 'I am so angry I am vomiting blood' may not actually represent hematemesis. Patients may not verbalize anxiety or doubts regarding their medical care in front of medical personnel, but will then not follow the treatments. This can be misinterpreted as patient non-compliance or insincerity. 'Saving face' may make it harder for patients to admit to having problems, especially concerning mental health or infertility issues. They may go as far as misrepresenting details of home remedies or hide details of visits to other healthcare providers. They may not want to question or disagree with the physician to their face, so they will not come back and will 'shop around' for another doctor or not take medication as prescribed. Furthermore, many Chinese still believe in traditional Chinese medical treatments, and a total disregard or lack of respect for these beliefs may lead to distrust.

Western methods of psychotherapy may not be received well; group teaching, support groups or therapy sessions are considered embarrassing. Confrontation may make patients uncomfortable though for the younger generation of Chinese immigrants, raising one's voice to a patient may generate a greater sense of authority, particularly by female healthcare providers. Open discussion and flexibility may go a long way in treating the Chinese patient, as it will with others.

Family members often want to stay with the hospitalized person continuously, providing all personal care. Hospitalizations can be frightening to individuals who are often fearful of spirits and ghosts, particularly at night. Family members should be made aware of the visiting hours of the hospital or special arrangements should be made to allow a family member to stay with the patient. Respect and obligation demand that children provide care for their parents.

Contraception and reproduction

Following the implementation of the 'one child' policy in China, contraceptive use and abortion practices have become quite commonplace. The Chinese generally avoid oral or hormonal contraception, but the intrauterine contraceptive device and tubal sterilization are acceptable.

Abortion. According to the accepted Confucian view, ensoulment of the fetus begins at the time of birth. A person is an entity that has a body or shape and psyche, and has rational, emotional and social-relational capacity. Therefore, a human embryo is not a person or a human life. Destroying an embryo, as well as abortion, is not considered as killing a person. However, patients who are practicing Buddhists may find abortion objectionable and incompatible with their beliefs of reincarnation (see Chapter 1).

Following the Communist Revolution in mainland China and its 'one child' policy, abortion has become a widely practiced form of contraception there. Gender selection, with a marked preference for male offspring, continues to be practiced in China. Chinese immigrants to the USA continue to terminate female fetuses, despite having the reproductive freedom to have more than one child. Some will go as far as elective chorionic villus sampling or prenatal sonography simply to determine the sex of the fetus.

Pregnancy and birth. Because of the importance of family honor in Chinese culture, children are highly valued. However, Asian women may seek prenatal care late during pregnancy or not at all, because of fear, cost and/or lack of need (pregnancy is not considered a illness, so why see a doctor?). Nevertheless, there are some unique folk religious practices among the Chinese related to childbirth; for example, lamb is avoided during pregnancy because it could cause the baby to have epilepsy (the pronunciation of the word 'lamb' is similar to the word for epilepsy in Chinese).

Many women are accompanied by their mother or mother-in-law during labor and birth, rather than by their husband, because this is considered women's work. It is acceptable for the new father to remain at work and not accompany his wife to the hospital, depending on the degree of acculturation. Women often prefer prenatal care from midwives and may prefer to assume the traditional squatting position during the birthing process. Asian women rarely cry or scream in pain or discomfort during labor to avoid bringing shame to the family. Pain and discomfort are considered a normal part of childbirth.

In Chinese folk religion, it is considered bad luck to speak about how beautiful a baby is or appear to prize the baby too highly, because the spirits may take the baby away by causing its death. Thus, parents may not exhibit 'usual' bonding behaviors such as cuddling or talking to the newborn. The mother will also avoid attracting the spirits to the infant by dressing the baby in old clothes and using nicknames that are negative or considered insulting by Western standards such as 'Stinky Butt' or 'Stupid Melon' to fool the spirits.

Women often follow the practice of a 30-day 'lying-in' period of confinement at home following birth, depending on the degree of acculturation. As the postpartum period may be considered a 'cold' state, bathing, shampooing the hair, cold liquids, cold air/drafts, exposure to the outdoors and exercise may be avoided. Ice packs to the perineum are likely to be refused. The woman will want to rest and stay warm. If the baby must stay in the hospital after the mother's discharge, women may not accompany the father to the hospital to visit the baby because of this lying-in period. Grandmothers, particularly the husband's mother, are often very involved with the new infant and the new mother's recovery. Their authoritative positions should be acknowledged when caring for the mother and during teaching sessions.

Mongolian spots are a common normal finding. They are bluish birthmarks on the backs and buttocks of newborns and cannot be washed off. Jaundice and higher bilirubin levels may be more prevalent among Chinese infants. Mild jaundice can be easily treated by exposing the newborn to sunlight, although taking the newborn outside is not permitted during the period of confinement.

During the postpartum period, 'cold' foods such as green vegetables, fruits, fruit juice, meats (excluding chicken) and fish are often avoided. Asian women do not usually drink iced water, so they should be offered warm liquids like water or tea. Special herbs specified for the postpartum period are usually added to soups. During the postpartum period, Chinese women may eat certain foods such as pigs' feet, sesame oil, ginger and other herbs to assist the removal of any placental remnants, to bring the body back into balance and to stimulate milk production. Consuming beef is usually avoided as it is thought to slow the healing process after birth.

Circumcision of male infants is considered barbaric by the Chinese and is generally not performed.

Breast-feeding. Mothers may be resistant to early breast-feeding, because colostrum is considered 'bad milk'. For this reason, the mother may insist on bottle-feeding the infant until her 'real milk' comes in.

Asian women are very concerned about modesty and should be provided with privacy while breast-feeding.

Concerns about family honor and a strong work ethic mean that working men do not take paternity leave and working women return to work as soon as their 30 days of confinement are over. In the USA, it is common for newborns as young as 3–6 months to be sent back to China to be raised by grandparents or extended families so that the parents can continue to work. This practice has led to a decrease in the number of Chinese women who choose to breast-feed their infants and reduced personal attachment to the newborn.

Sexuality

Chastity in unmarried men and women is highly valued. Premarital sex is considered strictly taboo. Chinese women generally are getting married later and having fewer children. In other parts of Asia, however, women tend to marry in their teens and have large families. Chinese women are generally very modest and therefore avoid gynecologic examinations, including prenatal care and cervical screening. This leads to high rates of cervical cancer and late prenatal care in China and immigrants of Chinese ancestry.

Homosexuality is not strictly forbidden by any of the Chinese religions, but is generally not openly spoken about.

Death

Many Chinese are reluctant to discuss issues regarding illness, death, end-of-life care or advance directives because they believe that if one speaks about something bad, it could occur (karma). Organ donation and autopsies are usually refused due to the influence of the Buddhist belief that if the body is cut, or organs or body parts are lost, the person will be incomplete during reincarnation.

Funerals are usually loud and noisy events to scare away evil spirits and to allow the family to wail. White is the color used at funerals and members of the mourning family will dress in white and white flowers will be used. Food and spirit money offerings are made, and the family altar is installed in the home. The Chinese prefer burials rather than the Buddhist practice of cremation. They consider the body and bones to have important powers that affect living family members. Traditional Chinese will consult feng-shui experts to determine the date, location and orientation of the corpse to bring the family good luck.

Stillbirth or pregnancy loss is not perceived to be as devastating as in Western culture where women consider the fetus as a person. Presenting the dead fetus to the mother, or taking photos or mementos of the fetus is not appreciated by the Chinese patient. Bereavement therapy and support groups are generally frowned upon.

Key points – Traditional Chinese Religion

- Traditional Chinese Religion is not an organized, unified system of beliefs but is underpinned by a series of philosophies emphasizing mind, body and social interactions.
- The practices and beliefs of practitioners of Chinese medicine are generally based on balances of 'hot' and 'cold', yin and yang, and harmony with the universe.
- Diets for diabetics may not be compatible with 'hot' and 'cold' foods, and consultation with a dietitian may be required.
- Self-administered aspects of Traditional Chinese Medicine (TCM) include meditation, exercise that cultivates the 'chi' (e.g. tai chi), general exercise and diet.
- Some aspects of TCM have been more widely incorporated into mainstream medical practice (e.g. acupuncture).
- Traditional Chinese and Western medical systems are very different, and patients may have difficulty expressing problems and following advice or treatment regimens.
- Patients of Chinese origin may try to avoid doctors, especially for preventive healthcare, and consultations may be very formal.
- Lower body weights and differences in metabolism should be taken into account when prescribing medication for Asian patients.
- The most senior male member of the family is usually the decision maker; some women may not be allowed to make healthcare decisions for themselves.

People belonging to a number of other religions have beliefs with specific healthcare implications. These religions include:

- Jehovah's Witnesses
- Seventh-day Adventists
- Rastafarians
- Mormons (The Church of Jesus Christ of Latter-day Saints).

Jehovah's Witnesses

Jehovah's Witnesses are part of a Christian sect that was founded in the USA in 1872 by Charles Taze Russell. The denomination spread to the UK in 1914 and is now an international religious organization with approximately 6.5 million members. Large numbers of Jehovah's Witnesses are also found in Brazil and Mexico. The name 'Jehovah's Witness' is derived from the bible in which God is referred to as Jehovah.

The Watchtower Bible and Tract Society of New York became a legal entity in 1881 and incorporated in 1884. The Jehovah's Witnesses are led by a governing body at their national headquarters, The Watchtower, in Brooklyn, New York, USA, while local congregations are typically located in buildings known as a 'Kingdom Hall'. Watchtower headquarters, and local congregations are run by church elders assisted by ministerial servants. Women have minimal leadership responsibilities, but participate in a large portion of preaching work.

The Jehovah's Witnesses are only one of several post-Reformation Protestant denominations that have flourished in the USA; others include Seventh-day Adventists, Baptists, Mormons (the Church of the Latter-day Saints) and Christian Scientists. The Witnesses are commonly known for their door-to-door preaching, refusal to accept blood transfusions, their religious magazines (*The Watchtower* and *Awake!*) and abstinence from celebrating birthdays and non-religious holidays. They are politically neutral and feel that God is their one true leader and not the national government. They refrain from singing the national anthem or saluting any flags that may represent 'false gods' or idols. They will pay state and federal taxes, but avoid voting in any political elections. They do, however, participate in international humanitarian relief efforts in order to promote their preaching to those less fortunate. Unlike other Christian denominations, Jehovah's Witnesses reject the concepts of the Holy Trinity, eternal torment in hell and the immortality of the soul. Their central belief is that Jesus Christ will have a second coming and rule the paradise on earth as its King.

The early leaders of this denomination were renowned for predicting the visible return of Christ in 1873, 1874 and 1975, and the end of the world (Armageddon) in 1914, which has now been revised to be 'imminent'.

Worship. Groups of Witnesses may congregate in a Kingdom Hall. Witnesses will attend the hall closest to them and one Kingdom Hall may serve several congregations and accommodate them at different times. Meetings are not necessarily structured services as in other Christian denominations, but may be bible study groups, talks from someone from the Watchtower Bible and Tract Society or a meeting of those engaged in door-to-door missionary work.

Scripture. Jehovah's Witnesses believe the Bible was inspired by God and is historically accurate. They have a very literal interpretation of the Bible, which has led to some of the stringent beliefs of their followers. The interpretation of the Bible is the responsibility of the Governing Body of the church.

Family. Marriages are required to be monogamous. Jehovah's Witness families are patriarchal; the husband is considered the final authority in all family decisions. Weddings and funerals are observed, but celebrations, such as birthdays, Thanksgiving or Christmas, or those that are considered nationalistic or false religion are avoided.

Dress. Modesty is encouraged in dress and grooming. Most of the men are clean shaven and wear white shirts with black ties, or plain suits. Otherwise, Jehovah's Witnesses do not wear any special garments that distinguish them.

Food and drink. Jehovah's Witnesses avoid eating meat that has not been properly bled because they believe it is wrong to eat blood. This has its origins in the Holy Bible (Genesis and Acts) in which followers are instructed not to eat meat that contains blood. Drunkenness is disapproved of as is alcohol which, like drug-taking, is seen as soiling the mind and making people slaves to a substance.

General health issues. Jehovah's Witnesses' literal interpretation of the Bible, which commands Christians to abstain from blood leads them to believe that accepting a blood transfusion will lead to their eternal damnation. The Governing Body has prohibited their followers from accepting transfusions of whole blood or the four primary components of blood: red blood cells, white blood cells, platelets and plasma. Jehovah's Witnesses have also been instructed not to donate or store their own blood for autologous transfusion because of the fear that any blood is impure after it has left the body.

As new medical technologies have developed, this fundamental prohibition requires additional scrutiny and is subject to personal interpretation. Followers of this denomination have been instructed by their leaders to use their 'bible-trained conscience' to make the appropriate personal medical decisions. It is important to recognize that not all Jehovah's Witnesses adhere to the same beliefs so it is important to have frank discussions alone with the individual patient without other family members in the room.

As well as considering the traditional transfusion of packed red blood cells (PRBCs), the Jehovah's Witness patient must now decide whether to accept other blood products such as human albumin in the setting of hypovolemia or clotting factors that are life saving in the case of hemophilia. For pregnant women, immunoglobulin and anti-D therapy (Rhogam™) for Rhesus-negative women may be a serious consideration to prevent Rhesus disease and stillbirth. Interferon is derived from white blood cells and a Jehovah's Witness suffering from multiple sclerosis may decline life-saving interferon therapy.

The Jehovah's Witness patient should also enter into detailed discussion with their healthcare provider, particularly in anticipation of major surgery or pregnancy, to determine whether alternatives to PRBC transfusion might be acceptable to their conscience and in their own interpretation of biblical scripture. Potentially controversial technologies include:

- cell savers
- hemodilution with autologous blood transfusion
- heart-lung bypass machine
- epidural blood patch
- dialysis
- plasmapheresis
- labeling or tagging blood cells for diagnostic testing.

Traditionally, children are considered minors and incapable of making competent medical decisions so parents have to make decisions on their behalf. However, courts in the USA, UK and Australia have made it clear that children requiring medically indicated blood transfusions or blood products can not be prohibited from receiving medical treatment based on parental religious belief.

Since the 1970s, the Watchtower Society has issued 'blood refusal cards' to its members. Most healthcare providers will abide by this advance directive under non-emergency situations. However, in an emergency, if there is any doubt as to the validity of the 'blood refusal card' and the patient is unconscious, physicians can err on the side of preserving life and administer life-saving blood products.

Contraception and reproduction. Jehovah's Witnesses avoid surrogate motherhood and reproductive technology techniques involving the use of donated eggs, sperm or embryos.

Abortion is considered murder and therefore strictly prohibited under all circumstances. The congregation is responsible for disciplining any members that violate church doctrines. Members are initially considered 'marked' and then 'disfellowshipped' or shunned by all fellow members. These decisions are made by a judicial committee of church elders in consultation with the Governing Body.

Pregnancy and birth. When a Jehovah's Witness woman presents for prenatal care, a complete blood count should be obtained and consideration given to commencing iron and folate supplementation. The goal should be to avoid anemia, which may be worsened at and following delivery. Erythropoietin may be considered for patients who are anemic.

If a woman is Rhesus negative, anti-D therapy (Rhogam™) may be indicated. As anti-D is a blood product, it may be declined by a Witness. Immunoglobulin infusion may be indicated for pregnant women with platelet or autoimmune disorders. If either these or any other blood products are to be considered, they must be discussed early on during the pregnancy and in full. If the mother declines, documentary evidence should be filed with her medical record.

Plans for management of the pregnant Jehovah's Witness patient should include delivery in a hospital setting with 24-hour in-house anesthesiology services and an open discussion of the patient's wishes with documentation of the discussion and a written plan in the event of a life-threatening hemorrhage.

Sexuality. Jehovah's Witnesses' views on sexuality are consistent with conservative Christian beliefs. Homosexuality and premarital sex are considered sins.

Death. Witnesses believe that when a person dies, their existence stops completely. They do not believe that a person has an immortal soul or in the concept of hell or a place where a person's soul may be tormented. However, a Witness may be remembered by God and eventually resurrected.

Seventh-day Adventists

The Seventh-day Adventist Church is a Christian Protestant denomination founded in the USA in the 1860s with the Bible as its holy book. The Church is named after the observance of the 'biblical Sabbath' on Saturday and the belief that Jesus Christ will soon return to earth ('Advent' or 'coming'). The faith is based on Christianity but differs on four main points: the Sabbath day is Saturday rather than Sunday; the status of Ellen White (see below); the beliefs regarding the millennium and the 'second coming'; and the concept of the heavenly sanctuary.

The foundations of the Church are the teachings of William Miller, an American preacher who preached that the 'second coming' or

Advent of Jesus was imminent. He predicted that Jesus would appear in 1844. Following the disappointment that this did not occur, many of his followers left the movement. Miller was followed by Ellen White, another preacher and prophet. White also taught that Jesus would return to earth, but that he would not do so until he had finished cleansing the 'most holy place' of the heavenly temple. She also taught that the Sabbath should be observed on a Saturday. Despite some early difficulties, the movement eventually declared itself a denomination in 1863.

It founded its first healthcare institution in 1866 and now runs several hundred medical facilities. The foundations of the Seventh-day Adventist healthcare tradition are based on 'wholeness' and the healing of mind, body and spirit, and the fact that Jesus ministered to the whole person. Health has both a missionary as well as an individual purpose for Adventists.

Seventh-day Adventists differ from other Christians in that they do not believe that people go to heaven or hell when they die, but that the dead remain unconscious until Christ returns to judge them. There is no concept of a surviving soul or spirit, but those who give their life to Christ may eventually be resurrected to an immortal life while sinners and non-believers will die for all eternity.

Worship. Adventist families come together on a Friday evening at the start of the Sabbath (sundown on Friday) and gather for a family meal. The period until sundown on a Saturday is regarded as a time for prayer, rest and the avoidance of secular reading or broadcasts. It may be used for visiting the sick and the salvation of souls but it is not a time for unnecessary work.

Diet. The Adventist lifestyle is simple, and maintenance of personal health is mentioned specifically in the doctrine. Rules about food laid down in the book of Leviticus in the Holy Bible are followed, similar to those of observant Jews. Many Adventists are vegetarian though this is not mandatory. If meat is eaten, it must be prepared according to biblical instructions similar to meat that is regarded as *kosher* for Jews. Pork products are not eaten.

The Adventists are responsible for an aspect of life taken for granted in many Western households – the breakfast cereal. John Harvey Kellogg, an Adventist preacher, invented cornflakes as a replacement for bacon and eggs.

Lifestyle. Adventists do not smoke, use recreational drugs or alcohol.

Sexuality. Sex outside marriage is forbidden. Young people are expected to take responsibility for avoiding sexual encounters, aided by their parents chaperoning them at meetings. Monogamous heterosexual marriage is the only acceptable form of sexual expression. Homosexuality is banned. Adventist ministers will not marry a couple unless both partners are Adventists themselves. Divorce is only permissible if one or both partner(s) has committed adultery, engaged in 'sexual perversion' or become a non-believer. The church will attempt to reconcile a couple before granting a divorce. In the case of a couple divorcing due to adultery or non-belief, the partner who has remained faithful may remarry, while the other partner may not for as long as their ex-partner lives.

Rastafarians

Rastafari is a young religion founded in Jamaica in the 1930s following the coronation of King Haile Selassie I in Ethiopia. King Selassie is known as 'the Conquering Lion of Judah' and the lion is the symbol of the faith. Rastafari began with the prophecy of Marcus Garvey, a political activist who wanted to improve the lives of fellow black citizens. He decreed that a 'black king shall be crowned, he shall be your redeemer' and shortly afterwards the coronation of King Selassie fulfilled the prophecy. Having started in Jamaica, the religion spread globally following the success of Bob Marley and his music in the 1970s.

    Central to Rastafari is the belief that black people are the chosen people of God and that their role has been suppressed by slavery and colonization. The movement's greatest concerns are the repatriation of black people to Africa and elevating the status of black people in society. Haile Selassie, though outside the religion, is considered as God. The holy book is the Holy Bible from which a number of practices are taken. These include the dietary laws as laid out in the Old Testament and abstention from alcohol. Clean and natural foods are preferred and meat, especially pork, is avoided.

The ritual use of marijuana is widespread as it is believed to enhance spiritual awareness. Rastafarians are forbidden to cut their hair (Old Testament law), and grow it and twist it into dreadlocks. With reference to the symbol of the faith – the lion – dreadlocks represent the lion's mane.

Rastafarians are opposed to abortion and contraception, and there are certain aspects of the faith that apply only to women. Although there are now more variable expressions of these rules, early adherents followed them more strictly. Women are regarded as Queens and their men as Kings. It is the duty of women to look after their Kings and they are regarded as subordinate. Women must keep the house and raise children. A woman must be faithful to her man and must not cook for him while menstruating. The use of contraception is prohibited as it is believed to be a tool developed by white people to suppress the development of the African population. Abortion is regarded as murder. Women also keep their hair long and in dreadlocks, but also cover their hair according to biblical teaching which states that women who pray with uncovered heads disgrace their husbands.

Mormons

The Church of Jesus Christ of Latter-day Saints was founded in the USA in the 19th century by Joseph Smith and its adherents are called Mormons. Mormons have been present in the UK since the early 1800s and there are currently 190 000 members in the UK.

The church is based in Salt Lake City, Utah, USA, where the church migrated under the new leadership of Brigham Young in 1847. The church headquarters consists of a large campus of awesome buildings, including the famous Tabernacle (which is closed to non-Mormon visitors) and the Convention Center (which is open to the public and helps to recruit new followers). The Mormon Tabernacle Choir is internationally renowned for its sheer size and the ability of all the voices to sing in harmony.

Mormons believe that the church is a restoration of the Church as conceived by Jesus and that other Christian churches have gone astray. Mormons believe that God has a physical presence, is married and can have children. They also believe that humans can become gods in the afterlife.

The Mormons use the Old and New Testaments of the Bible, but also worship in the *Book of Mormon*, a 'lost book' of the bible which chronicles other religious figures who traveled to the New World (South America) around the time of Jesus Christ. The Mormons are led by a single Prophet that is elected by a council of Bishops when a previous Prophet has died. All prophets have been men since Brigham Young, the original Prophet.

Their members are expected to preach and proselytize. Their recruitment of new followers has been extremely successful, and new Mormon Churches are being constructed across the USA, even in Chinatown areas. They are clean cut; the men are usually seen wearing black suits, white shirts and black ties, and the women dress conservatively.

Mormons have a strong focus on family life. They have large families of five children or more. Some Mormon sects practice polygamy so that they can have large families. Contraception is accepted and is up to the individual. Mormons are strongly opposed to abortion, but it may be justified in exceptional circumstances. They do not smoke, drink alcohol, gamble, drink tea or coffee, use illicit drugs and are opposed to pornography and sex outside heterosexual marriage.

Mormons prefer to bury rather than cremate their dead. Mormons believe in life after death and that a death is a temporary separation from a person whom they will meet again. In this way, grief is tempered with the hope of meeting again.

Fasting is a regular feature of Mormon life and church members will go without two consecutive meals on the first Sunday of each month. The money that would have been spent on food is given to the church. On these particular Sundays, the Mormon community will come together for fasting and testimony meetings. In line with other religions, fasting is designed to assist prayerful reflection and focus on spiritual matters.

Key points – Other religions

- Jehovah's Witnesses are prohibited from accepting blood transfusions or any blood products.
- Seventh-day Adventists promote a healthy lifestyle and sponsor healthcare centers worldwide based on 'wholeness' and the healing of mind, body and spirit.
- Ritual use of marijuana is widespread among Rastafarians, as it is believed to enhance spiritual awareness.
- Fasting is a regular feature of Mormon life.

Fasting

Fasting is practiced by members of a number of faiths for variable lengths of time and with variable frequency. In the context of religious belief, fasting is believed to enhance the ability to focus on prayer and spiritual purification.

There are a variety of interpretations of fasting. Christians, for example, may fast overnight so that the stomach is empty on partaking of the Eucharist at Mass early in the morning. Followers of other religions may fast during the day and allow a meal at sundown. Some fasting rules allow water, others do not.

In general, fasting is safe. Evidence demonstrates that 1 year after renal transplantation, fasting has no detrimental effect on an individual. Furthermore, the quantities of milk produced by breast-feeding women are not significantly reduced. Possibly the greatest potential medical consequences of fasting may be seen in observant Muslims undertaking the fast for the Holy month of Ramadan (see Chapter 4) when complete fasting from dawn until dusk is observed for a month.

Potential risks. A patient altering a medication schedule without advice has obvious potential undesirable or even dangerous consequences. For example, taking all the medication for a day in a single dose rather than in divided doses may lead to toxicity, especially in the elderly, and short-acting medication taken once daily will not have any effect for the greater part of the day. In particular, patients with diabetes need clear advice to avoid complications (see below). Mild dehydration with symptoms of progressive lassitude and headaches is common, especially if fasting takes place during the summer and for many days at a time.

Changes to medication. The physician and patient should assess the safety of fasting by taking into consideration the environmental, occupational and individual health factors. Patients on long-term oral medications can usually have their treatment changed to an alternative that is acceptable and which, if effective, can be continued after the fasting period. Short-acting treatments taken several times a day often have a long-acting equivalent (e.g. modified release nitrates or analgesics). Long-acting inhaled therapy for asthma is also available.

Changing the route of administration may circumvent the issue of oral medication. Some medicines are available in sublingual, transdermal or rectal forms. However, many patients dislike suppositories and this should be discussed before they are prescribed.

Diabetes. Patients with diabetes need to be clear about alterations to their normal regimen in order to fast safely (Table 9.1). Although fasting poses potential complications in diabetes, they seem to be uncommon in practice.

TABLE 9.1

Advice for patients with diabetes during fasting

Diet-controlled diabetes

- Make the pre-dawn meal the major meal of the day
- Space other meals evenly over the non-fasting period

Oral medication

- If on a single daily dose, take the medication with the sunset meal
- If medication is taken more than once daily, switch the morning dose and any midday dose with the evening (sunset) dose

Insulin-dependent diabetes

- Fasting should be avoided in those prone to wide swings in blood sugar or ketoacidosis
- If on a once daily regimen, change to twice daily
- If on a twice daily regimen, take a third or a half of the normal morning dose and the usual evening dose

Adapted from Fazel M. Medical implications of controlled fasting. *J Roy Soc Med* 1998:91;260–3.

Female circumcision

Female circumcision or female genital mutilation (FGM) is not encouraged by Islamic religious doctrine. However, it is practiced in over 30 countries in Africa, mostly those with Muslim majorities, and to a much lesser extent in the Middle East. The reasons given include prevention of masturbation and female promiscuity, promotion of female hygiene and fertility, and preservation of virginity. Furthermore, in some communities, an uncircumcised woman has no chance of marriage, may be seen as promiscuous and is therefore socially unacceptable.

FGM may take several forms according to the traditions of a particular community, but commonly involves excision of the prepuce, clitoris and labia minora. Infibulation or 'pharaonic circumcision' involves removing all external genitalia and suturing the sides of the vulva together, leaving only a small hole through which urine and menstrual blood may escape.

The procedures are usually carried out in childhood, from 4 years of age upwards, without anesthetic, by female elders of the community but can take place at any time from infancy to adolescence.

The physical and emotional health risks both in the short and long term are considerable. Bleeding and infection present immediate risks. Recurrent urinary tract infections are not uncommon as the healing process may inhibit the passing of urine and encourage urinary stasis. Once healed, the opening of the vagina may be so small as to prohibit sexual intercourse and circumcised women may require formal reversal of circumcision before and/or episiotomy at the time of vaginal delivery to permit childbirth.

In many countries, including the UK and USA, it is illegal to undertake or abet female circumcision either at home or abroad. In order to circumvent this legislation, parents may take their children abroad 'on holiday' to their home countries. In the UK, any professional in contact with female children whom they believe to be at risk of being circumcised is obliged to report any concerns or suspicions to the appropriate authorities.

Key points – General health issues

- Fasting is subject to a variety of interpretations, but is generally safe for most patients.
- Patients taking medication, particularly those with diabetes, must be given clear advice to avoid complications.
- Mild dehydration is common in fasting patients, especially in the summer.
- Female circumcision is widely practiced in Africa and may take several forms.
- The physical and emotional health risks of female circumcision are considerable, both in the short and long term.
- In many countries, it is illegal to undertake or abet female circumcision.

Useful resources

British Broadcasting Corporation. www.bbc.co.uk/religion (Good, accessible coverage of a wide variety of religions. There are links to other websites and useful telephone numbers for contacts regarding many of the listed religions. It also has a calendar of festivals, holy days and other useful dates for all the major faiths.)

Koenig HG. *Sprituality in Patient Care: Why, When, How and What?* 2nd edn. West Conshohocken, PA: Templeton Foundation Press, 2007. (A book for the caregiver, which explores how to integrate a patient's notion of their own spirituality into healthcare.)

Morgen Krueger Ltd. www.interfaithcalendar.org (An interfaith calendar of the world's major faiths.)

Neuberger E, Neuberger J. *Caring for Dying People of Different Faiths.* 3rd edn. Oxford: Radcliffe Publishing, 2004. (A more detailed look at this rite of passage from various major world faith perspectives.)

Orchard H, ed. *Spirituality in Healthcare Contexts.* London: Jessica Kingsley Publishers, 2001. (A book mainly designed for those providing spiritual care in the context of healthcare, but also an interesting look at the topic of religion and medicine from another perspective).

Sheikh A, Gatrad AR, eds. *Caring for Muslim Patients.* 2nd edn. Oxford: Radcliffe Publishing, 2007. (An excellent, comprehensive text, which covers, in detail, a wide range of subjects relating to the emotional and physical health of Muslim patients.)

Spitzer J. *Caring for Jewish Patients.* Oxford: Radcliffe Publishing, 2003. (A book devoted to aspects of Jewish culture and belief that may impact on the care of a person from that faith.)

Index

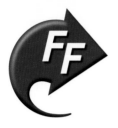
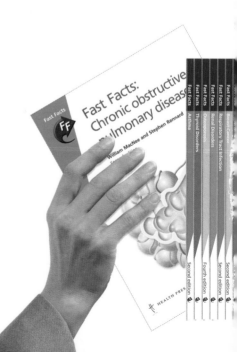